VEGAN MEAL PREP
for Beginners

Ready-to-Go Meals for Weight Loss
and Healthy Eating.
An Easy Guide with 4 Weekly Plans
and Vegan Recipes.

Mark Power

Table of Contents

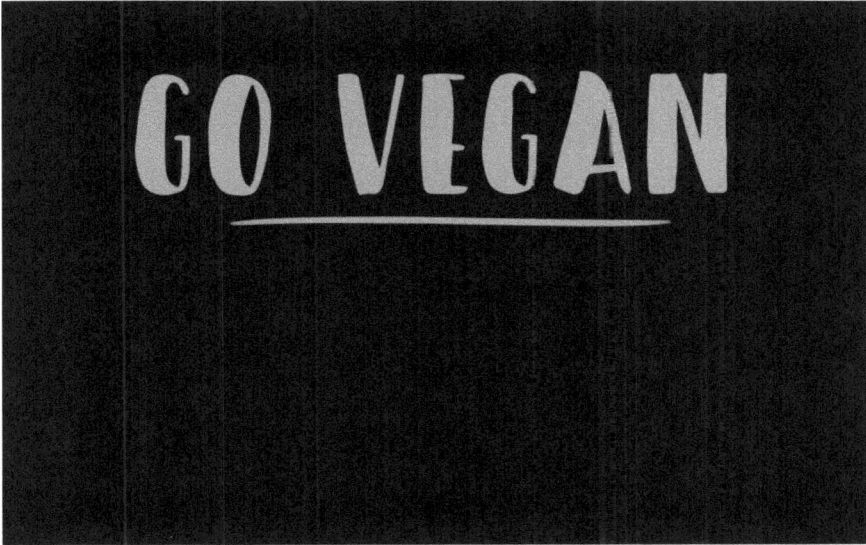

Congratulations on purchasing *Vegan Meal Prep for Beginners* and thank you for doing so.

The following chapters will discuss everything that you need to know in order to get started with the vegan diet, and how to add in some of the meal prep parts that we need as well. There are so many things out there to enjoy when it comes to following the vegan diet, and it is one of the best dietary choices to go with when you want to lose weight and improve your health. But it is sometimes hard to stick with it and be prepared. And that is why we will introduce the idea of meal planning into this and learn how we can combine the vegan diet with meal planning tips to make life easier.

The beginning of this diet plan is going to take a look at the vegan diet and what it is all about. We will start out with some of the many health benefits of this diet plan and why so many people want to jump on and learn more about how to follow it easily. We can then move on to learning more about the foods that are allowed and the ones that you should avoid in order to get results with this diet plan.

Once we know a bit more about the vegan diet and what it is all about, it is time for us to jump in and learn more about meal prepping. We are going to take a look at what meal prepping is and some of the benefits of using this, how to prepare your kitchen so it is ready for some of the meal prepping and for he vegan diet in general, and then we will talk about how you can find the best meals and recipes for your needs when it comes to the vegan diet so you can enjoy your meal plan as well.

From there it is time to take a look at some of the other exciting things that we are able to do when it comes to preparing for the vegan diet with some meal planning. We will look at how meal prepping can help you lose weight and reach all of your health goals, how to organize your shopping list, and some of the basics of the meal plan to help you get started, including four weeks of meal prep ideas to help you get going on this plan.

The end of this guidebook is going to take a look at the recipes that you are able to use when it comes to working on this kind of diet plan. There are so many delicious vegan recipes that you are able to work with. We will take a look at those that work for breakfast, lunch, dinner, and dessert so that you can make some of the best recipes for your needs and ensure that you are able to really get healthy and ready to handle your meal planning goals in no time.

There are a lot of benefits of the vegan diet, and when you combine it together with some of the benefits that come with the meal planning that we will talk about in this guidebook, you are sure to see a lot of results in the process. It is a fast and easy way to make sure that you are getting all of your nutrients and can make weight loss and good health fall into your grasp faster than ever before. When you are ready to get started with how to use meal planning to help with following the vegan diet, make sure to check out this guidebook to help.

Last but not least important, avoiding animal products is one of the most obvious ways you can take a stand against animal cruelty and animal exploitation everywhere.

There are plenty of books on this subject on the market, thanks again for choosing this one! Every effort was made to ensure it is full of as much useful information as possible, please enjoy it!

PART 1

ALL ABOUT THE VEGAN DIET

Chapter 1 - The Many Benefits of the Vegan Diet

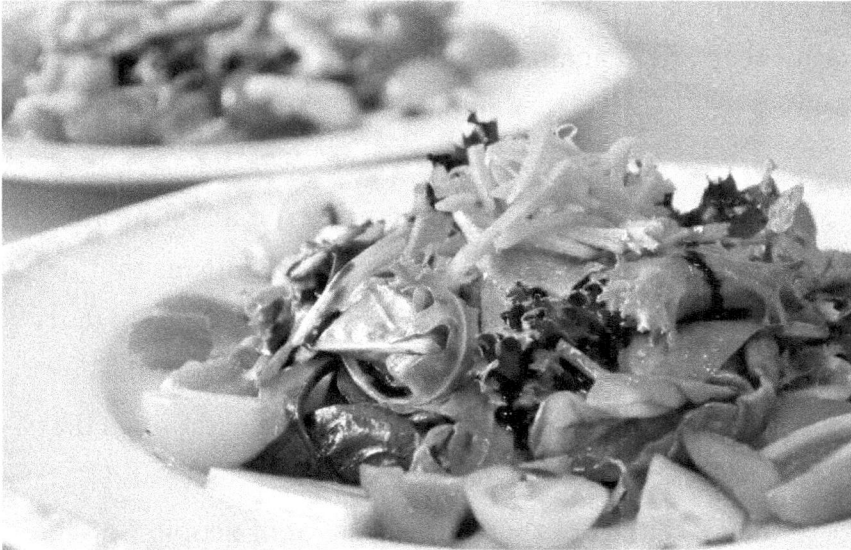

There are a lot of diet plans out there that we can choose to follow. Some are going to be low fat and encourage us to eat lots of healthy carbs and fruits and vegetables. Some are going to be low carb and will take it the completely other way and have you cut out the carbs and ramp up the number of fats you eat. Then there are those that are more about getting lots of protein into your day and that can be a great option as well. And then there are some diets that are more about just having moderation on all of the foods you eat and don't lean too much one way or another.

But the diet plan that we are going to discuss in this guidebook is known as the vegan diet. This is a healthy diet that is good for helping people to lose weight and provides us with a ton of other health benefits in the process as well. it can help us to maintain a healthy heart, fight against certain types of cancers and is good for fighting against type two diabetes.

Basically, the vegan diet is all about cutting out all of the animal sources of food, and any animal products. This means that not only are things like meat out, but eggs and many types of dairy are going to be restricted as well. many people go on this diet because it helps them to eliminate some of the bad things that are in their dies and can make it easier to lose weight and improve their health. But there are also a lot of people who like to go on this kind of diet because of ethical reasons or because they want to keep things better for the environment.

There are actually a lot of benefits that you are able to enjoy when it comes to a vegan diet and following it for your health. Some of the best benefits that you can enjoy when it comes to the vegan diet will include:

It Is Rich in Nutrients

If you switch from the typical American diet over to a vegan diet, it is true that you are going to eliminate a lot of the animal and meat products. This is going to lead you to rely more on some of the other foods out there. If you are working with the whole-foods version of the vegan diet, the replacements that you will work with will take the form of whole grains, nuts and seeds, peas beans, fruits, and vegetables. Since these foods are going to really take up a big proportion of the vegan diet compared to what we see in the typical American diet, they are going to ensure that we take in a higher amount of some of the beneficial nutrients that our body needs.

For example, several studies have shown that these kinds of diets are going to provide the body with more antioxidants and more fiber than the traditional diet. They are also going to be higher in things like vitamins A, C, and E along with folate, magnesium, and potassium, all of which are good for us. We have to keep in mind though that not all of the versions of the vegan diet are going to be equal. For example, some of the vegan diets out there are not going to be well-planned and will not provide us with the right amounts of essential fatty acids, zinc, iodine, calcium, iron or vitamin B12. This is why it is important to stay away from the fast-food or nutrient-poor options for the vegan diet. They may be considered vegan, but this does not mean that they are good for you. You should base the diet around whole and nutrient-rich plants and fortified foods. You can even consider starting with a supplement like vitamin B12 to help at the beginning of this diet.

Helps Get Rid of Extra Weight

There are a lot of people who are deciding to turn to a diet that is based on plants to help them to get rid of their extra weight, and there is a lot of good reason for that. There have been a number of observational studies that show how most vegans, as least the ones who follow the diet in the proper manner, are going to be thinner and have a lower body mass index compared to those who are not vegans. In addition, a few randomized controlled studies are able to report that these vegan diets are going to be more effective for weight loss than any of the diets that were compared to them.

In one of these studies, it showed that the vegan diet helped those who followed it lose 9.3 pounds more than those who were in a control diet of another sort over an 18-week study period. What was interesting was that the ones who followed the vegan diet lost more weight than those who had to follow the calorie-restricted diets, even though the vegan groups did not count calories and were allowed to eat until they felt full.

What is more with this is that in a study that compared the weight loss effects that show up in five different diets, it was found that both the vegetarian and the vegan diets were just as well-accepted as some of the results in the standard Western diets and the semi-vegetarian diets. Even when they were not following these diets 100 percent, the vegan and the vegetarian groups were still able to lose more weight than those who went on one of the standard Western diets as well.

Helps to Lower Blood Sugar Levels

Going vegan could help out those who are suffering from type 2 diabetes and declining kidney function. In fact, vegans are going to have lower levels of blood sugars, a higher sensitivity to insulin, and their risk of developing type 2 diabetes in the first place can go down by up to 78 percent. Studies even show that the vegan diet is able to lower the levels of blood sugars in those who are diabetic more than some of the best-known diets out there, even compared to the diet recommended by the American Diabetes Association.

In one study that was done on this, about 43 percent of the participants who were following a vegan diet were able to reduce their dosage of medications that they used to lower blood sugars, while only 26 percent of those who were on the diet recommended by the ADA was able to do the same. Some other studies report that diabetics who substitute meat for plant protein may be able to reduce their risk of poor kidney functioning as well.

If you are someone who is dealing with the higher levels of blood sugars, then the vegan diet is going to be the right one for you to use as well. it is simple and it is one of the best ways to get your levels of blood sugars down and to a more manageable amount in no time.

May Be Able To Protect Against Cancers

According to the World Health Organization, about one-third of all cancers can be prevented by factors that are within our control and one of these is the diet that we follow. For example, eating legumes on a regular basis may be enough to help reduce our risk of colorectal cancer by up to 18 percent. Research also suggests that eating at least seven portions of fresh fruits and vegetables per day may help to lower our risk of dying from cancer up to 15 percent.

As we can imagine, vegans are generally going to eat more legumes, fruits, and vegetables compared to those who do not follow this kind of eating plan. This could help to explain why a recent review that went over 96 studies found that vegans are able to have a 15 percent lower risk of developing or dying from cancer. What's more, vegan diets are going to contain more soy products, which is believed to offer some protection against breast cancer.

Avoiding some of the animal products that are found in the traditional diet could be what is going to help reduce the risk of colon cancers, breast cancers, and even prostate cancers. This could be due to the fact that vegan diets are going to be without smoked or processed meats or other types of meats that are cooked at high temperatures. Which could promote some types of cancers? Vegans are also going to avoid a lot of dairy products which are thought to increase the risk of prostate cancer.

Lowers Your Risk of Heart Disease

Eating fresh fruits, vegetables, legumes, and fiber is going to be linked to a lower risk of heart disease overall. All of these are going to be eaten in a relatively large amount when we are on a vegan diet that has been planned out well. Observational studies that compare vegans and the general public found that those who were vegan had about a 75 percent lower risks of developing high blood pressure at some point. Vegans could also have up to a 42 percent lower risk from dying of heart disease as well.

In addition to all of this, there are more randomized and controlled studies out there that show us how the vegan diet is going to be more effective when it comes to reducing LDL cholesterol, reducing blood sugar levels, and even the total cholesterol levels of those who follow them compared to any of the other diets we look at. This can be really beneficial to the health of the heart since reducing all three of these things can reduce your risk of developing heart disease at some point by up to 46 percent.

Can Reduce Arthritis Pain

There are even a few studies out there that have taken a look at how the vegan diet has such a positive effect on people who suffer from various forms of arthritis in their lives. One study randomly took 40 arthritis participants and had them either continue to follow their traditional omnivorous diet or switched some of them to a plant-based and whole-food vegan diet. Both had to follow it for six weeks total.

Those who went on the vegan diet reported that they had higher energy levels and a better general functioning compared to those who didn't make any changes to their diet. Then there were two other studies that took the time to investigate the effects on a probiotic-rich, raw food vegan diet on symptoms of rheumatoid arthritis. Both of these reported that those who went in the vegan group experienced much better improvements in a lot of symptoms including morning stiffness, joint swelling, and pain compared to those on a traditional kind of diet.

As we can see, there are a lot of benefits that come with following this kind of diet plan, and pretty much anyone is able to benefit from using it for their own needs. With the right kinds of foods, and making sure that we don't fall into the trap of assuming that just because it says it is vegan doesn't mean it is a good option to eat, we will be able to eat a much healthier lifestyle that is good for us.

How Do I Follow the Vegan Diet?

Now that we have had a chance to take a look at some of the benefits that we need to work with when it comes to choosing the vegan diet, it is now time to take a look at some of the steps that we are able to take in order to stick with this diet. We already know some of the basics, such as those on this diet are not allowed to eat meats, but we have to remember that animal products, or anything that comes from an animal, like milk and eggs, had to be avoided as well.

We are going to take a look at some of the foods that you are able to eat on this kind of diet plan first. There are a lot of great tasting foods that you are going to love and can really spice up your meals, though it may seem like you are limited when you first get started. Some of the different foods that you are able to consume when you are on the vegan diet will include:

1. **_Legumes:_** This would include lots of different foods like lentils, beans, and peas. These are going to provide us with a lot of beneficial compounds from plants and other nutrients that can keep us nice and healthy as long as we need it.

2. **_Nuts and nut kinds of butter:_** You will find that the unroasted and unblanched versions are going to be the best. You should also stay away from those that are salted or have extra things on them. These means don't go out and buy the candied ones or the ones covered in chocolate and assume you are getting all of the good benefits.

3. **_Tempeh, seitan, and tofu:_** These are some of the best options to go with when it comes to finding lots of protein on this diet. Since you have to kick out eggs, fish, meat, and poultry on this one, you will find that adding in the three options above can be a good choice to still get your protein and other nutrients.

4. **_Seeds:_** these do have some of the protein and the omega-3 fatty acids that are hard to get on this diet plan along with some of the other nutrients that your body may be needed at the time. You will want to stick with some of

the options like flaxseeds, chia, and hemp to get the most benefits.

5. ***Nutritional yeast:*** This is another way to add in a bit more protein to any of the vegan dishes that you work with. And it can kind of add in a cheese flavor to these dishes as well. if you are able to find a variety that is fortified with B12, then go with this option as well.

6. ***Plant yogurts and milk that are fortified with calcium can be good options as well:*** these are going to ensure that you are able to get in all of the calcium that you need. And there are a lot of different varieties so you are sure to find the one that works the best for your needs.

7. ***Fruits and vegetables:*** both are going to be awesome foods to go with to help increase your intake of nutrients. You can go with a lot of different types of these to keep yourself healthy and provide more of the nutrients that our bodies need to be strong and do well.

8. ***Whole grains and cereals.*** These are going to be good sources of some of the minerals that we need along with the B-vitamins, iron, fiber, and the complex carbs that we need to make it through the day. There are a lot of options that come with this one; you just need to take the time to pick out the wholesome ones, and not the baked goods or other processed pieces of bread, to keep yourself healthy on this diet plan.

Now that we know a bit more about the foods that we are allowed to have on the vegan diet, it is time to take a look at some of the foods that we should avoid instead. Vegans are going to make it their goal to avoid eating any animal foods, and they will need to avoid foods that contain ingredients that come from an animal as well. this is going to limit a few of the foods that you may be used to enjoying on a traditional diet. But these are taken away to help improve your health, along with a few other reasons as well. some of the foods that we need to avoid when it comes to following the vegan diet includes:

1. *Poultry and meat:* This is going to include any of the meat sources that you may have had in the past. The obvious choices like beef, organ meat, chicken, goose, turkey, and more all need to be taken off. If it comes from an animal, you are not supposed to eat it on this diet plan.

2. *Animal-based ingredients:* These are a bit harder to work with or recognize, but they are based on animals and those products so they are important to kick out as well. you will want to avoid things like shellac, gelatin, albumen from egg whites, lactose, whey, and casein for example.

3. *Fish and seafood:* These are going to fit into the category of meat products as well, so anything that you

are able to catch and eat from the sea, you will need to avoid when you go on this kind of diet plan as well.

4. **Bee products:** Any of the products that come from bees needs to be avoided when you are on this kind of diet as well. this means that things like the royal jelly, bee pollen, and honey all need to be taken from the list as well.

5. **Dairy:** This is going to include lots of different options that we may be used to having on this kind of diet. It, of course, means that we need to avoid the milk and cheeses, though there are some vegan alternatives that you can choose to enjoy, and we also need to avoid options like ice cream, butter, yogurt, and cream.

6. **Eggs:** And finally, we need to be careful about eggs as well. there are ways to make your own eggs in this kind of diet plan, but you should not eat the traditional eggs or you will not be following this diet plan. Any eggs that come from options like fish, chickens, quails or ostriches should be avoided.

Following the vegan diet is going to be a little bit different than we may be used to working with in the past and with our traditional diets, but it is one of the best choices that you can make for your overall health and well-being as well. if you are worried about following this kind of plan, we will go through and talk about some of the meal prepping things that you can do to make it easier as we go through this guidebook. This will ensure that you are able to really get in control over the process and that you will not feel like you are drowning or not able to keep up as you go through this process.

CHAPTER 2 - ALL ABOUT MEAL PREPPING

Now it is time for us to dive into some of the basics that come with meal prepping and why this is going to be the best thing for you when you first get started on the vegan diet. When you were reading through some of the different rules and guidelines of the vegan diet, it may have seemed a bit overwhelming at first. But when we are able to add in a little bit of meal planning to the mix, it makes it a whole lot easier. We won't have to struggle each night to throw things together and worry about what recipes we will create and use. We can instead focus on doing this all at once and just take the rest of the week off to relax. With that in mind, let's dive into some of the basics of meal prepping and how it can be so good for the vegan diet.

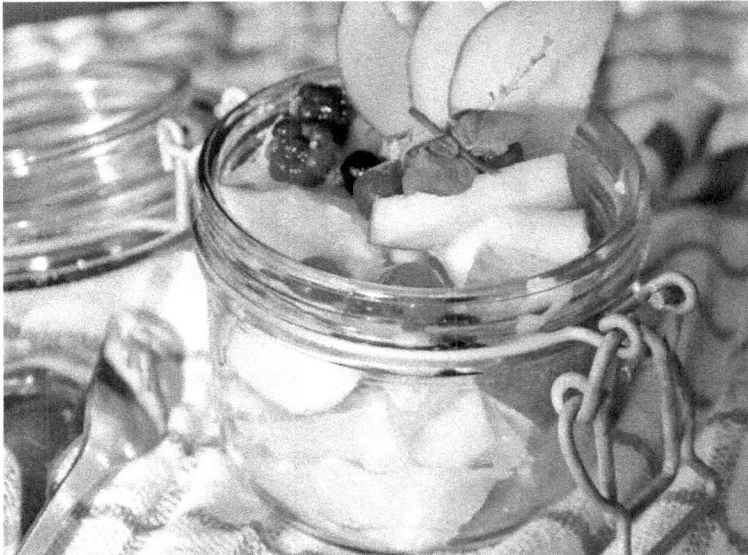

The Different Ways to Meal Prep

Many people make the assumption that there is only one way that they can meal prep, and if that method doesn't work for them then there is no point in even trying at all. They don't realize that there are actually quite a few ways that we can work on meal prepping, and we are going to take some time to look at some of the methods that we can use. Some of the most popular methods of meal prepping that are out there that you can choose will include:

1. The meals that are made ahead of time. These are going to be when we cook up full meals ahead of time and then we put them in the freezer or fridge. Then, when it is time to use them, we just have to heat them back up. This can be really helpful when it comes to dinner when everyone is tired and hungry. You can put one in the oven and then cook it up without having to do all of the other steps.

2. Batch cooking. This is when you will make a large batch of a specific recipe and then split it into smaller portions to be frozen and eaten over the next few months. You may make a really big lasagna and ten split it into three or four and have them ready when it works for you.

3. Meals that are individually portioned. Preparing fresh meals and then portioning them into some individual grab and go portions to be put in the fridge and then eaten over a few days is another option. This can be helpful to keep you on track when you are getting some lunches ready to go for your needs.

4. Ready to cook ingredients: This is when you prepare all of the ingredients that you need for a specific number of meals ahead of time. You will still cook the meals along the way, but the ingredients will be ready so you can just throw them all together when it is time and get it done quickly.

The method that is going to work the best for you is really going to depend on your own daily routine and your overall goals. If you are trying to make your morning a bit easier, for example, then preparing some breakfasts ahead of time may be the best way to help out. But some families like to have batch cooked meals in the freezer so they are all set to go when they are limited on time in the evenings. It is possible to do some mixing and matching when it comes to doing any of the meal prepping options above, so you are able to choose the one that will work the best for you.

Picking the Right Variety of Meals

The next thing that we need to consider is how to pick out the right variety of meals. Figuring out how many meals to make and what you would like to include in each of the meals is going to be tricky. The best way to plan ahead for this is to decide which meals would be the best to focus on, and which of the methods of meal prepping seems to be the best. Then you can check out your calendar to see how many of each meal you would like to prepare ahead of time for the upcoming week. We also need to remember to account for some of the situations where we may go out to eat for dates, client dinners, or just hanging out with friends.

When we select which meals to make, it is best to start with a limited number of recipes that we already know. This is going to ease our transition into meal planning. With this said, we need to try not to pick out just one recipe for the whole week. This may sound like a nice idea and like it will make life easier, but in reality, it is going to lead to boredom and will lack some of the nutrients that your body needs. It can also make it so that you are less likely to stick with the meal plan that you have.

Each person is going to be a bit different from what they would like to do here. Some will like to pick a large variety of meals and will constantly switch them out, and others are happy with sticking to a few of the same meals to keep it simple and because they know what they like. Both of these are going to work well when you handle meal planning; you just need to know which one you want to use and which one is the right choice for your needs. Don't sell yourself short on meals though if you are someone who likes a lot of variety because this is definitely something that we can do when working with the idea of meal planning and all that goes with it.

The Benefits of Meal Planning

Now we need to take a look at some of the best reasons and benefits as to why we would want to work with meal planning in the first place. Isn't it just fine to make the meals as you go and not have to worry about being organized and have it all together? There are a lot of people who choose to work with regular cooking and without doing meal planning, and that is fine to go with if it is your choice. But there are a ton of benefits that come with meal planning, and we need to take a look at a few of them.

The first benefit is that it is going to take away some of the indecision. There is nothing more frustrating than opening up all of the cupboards in your kitchen to see what is there. You wait for inspiration and ideas on what to cook, but there is nothing that stands out. Indecision is going to waste time, and if you can't figure it out, then you end up eating out and wasting money. When you have a meal plan, it is easier to go on autopilot and you will already have all of the ingredients, and even some of the meals that you need done.

You will also find that meal planning is going to lead to fewer bad choices. When you do not have a plan for your meals, it is going to lead us to make a lot of bad choices in what we will eat. Take out and ready meals are going to be quick and easy, and they can turn into habits if we are not that careful. And these are not healthy, even if they say they are vegan and can hit at your wallet as well.

Meal planning is going to help to remove the need to make these choices when you are tired or hungry, and when you are able to plan ahead of time, with a clear head, you will find that it is easier to make plans that have healthier foods with them. You can add in a few treats and a few extras for fun, but you will find that overall, meal planning takes out the bad choices and helps you to do a lot better.

Have you ever found yourself looking back at some of the meals and things that you have eaten and then you realize that you have been eating something that is pretty similar each night? This is not all that bad, but when you add in some meal planning you will find that it is easier to balance out your foods and you can actually get more variety into some of the meals that you are eating. This can make them more exciting and ensures that it is easier to stick with the vegan diet.

There is also the benefit that this kind of prepping is going to help you to reduce the amount of food that you waste and it can help you to save money. If you are able to create your meal plans and use your food in a wise manner, then you will naturally start to see a reduction in the amount of food that you are wasting. Buying only what is needed for your meals, and those are the ones that you already planned out, and not being swayed by offers that have nothing to do with what you want, can help you to save a lot of money over time.

Overall, working with meal planning is going to make your life a whole lot easier. It takes a bit of work and dedication, but you are going to love it when you can just go to the store and only get the items that you need. And it is even more fun when you are able to pull out the meal at the right time to eat, and all you have to do is heat it up without having to worry about cooking and preparing it all at that time. Get ready for the vegan diet, and your weekly routine, to get a lot easier.

How to Cut Down on Cooking Time

Even those who are big fans of meal prepping are not going to be that fond of cooking and spending hours in the kitchen to get this done. But we do need to spend at least a bit of time in the kitchen to get all of this done and make things easier during the week. Some of the steps that we are able to take to get our cooking time down as much as possible include:

1. *Stick with a schedule that is consistent.*

Meal prepping is going to work the best when you can still stick to a regular schedule. Knowing what you are going to get at the grocery store and how to prep all of your meals is going to keep you in a good routine and can make it easier. For example, you could choose to reserve Sunday morning to go grocery shopping and then have Monday for making lunches for the whole week. You can choose which schedule you want to go with but pick out one and stick with it to ensure that you can get in a good groove and that you will not feel overwhelmed all of the time with it.

2. Pick out a good combination of routines to do this with.

Picking out the right combination of recipes is going to ensure that you are a bit more effective in the kitchen. To save time, select recipes that have different methods of cooking. If you have too many recipes that all need the same appliance, you will not be able to prepare as many recipes at a time because they will have to wait for one another. This is going to be really important when you are trying to work with some make-ahead meals or when you do any kind of batch cooking.

3. Organize your prep and cook times.

If you think of your workflow ahead of time, it can really make things easier in the kitchen. To help you to organize your prep and cook times, you need to start out with the recipe that will take the longest amount of time to cook. This could be something like an oven meal or soup. Once you have that meal going, move on to the rest. Reserve all of the cold meals to do last because you can make them while the others are cooking.

You can even cut down on the cooking and prep time when you check the ingredients before you start. If you see that two or three of the recipes need diced onions, for example, you can just go through and chop out all that you need ahead of time without the worry.

4. *Make a shopping list.*

Spending time at the store can be a big waste of time. To cut down on how much time you are at the store, you can keep a detailed grocery list that is organized based on the departments of the supermarket. This is going to prevent issues with doubling back to a section that you already visited, and can speed up some of the time you spend at the store. You should also try to limit the shopping to just once a week and use the grocery delivery service to help spend fewer times hopping. This can also be a good way to cut down on your grocery bill as well.

How to be Successful with Meal Prepping

Getting a whole week's worth of meals, and sometimes more can seem like a daunting task to get started, especially when you are just beginning or you are trying to work with a vegan diet. The good news is that there are a lot of ways that we are able to make this a bit easier. Some of the simple steps that you are able to follow in order to be successful with meal prepping includes:

1. Select the right meal prep method of choice: This can also be a combination of methods and should be based on your own nutrition goals and your lifestyle.

2. Stick to a schedule: Pick one day each week that you want to do all of the meal planning, look for all of the groceries and cook.

3. Pick the right number of meals: You have to keep in mind your own personal calendar and the meals from restaurants that you have planned out for the week.

4. Select the recipes that you are right for you. Keep out an eye for variety and preparation methods. When you start out, it is usually best to just use some of the recipes you already know how to work with.

5. Try to find ways to reduce the time you spend on grocery shopping. Make a list that is as organized as possible or even work with shopping for your groceries online.

6. Send a little less time in the kitchen. You can choose which meals you would like to cook first and base this on the amount of time that it takes to cook those meals.

7. Store the meals. You need to work with some of the safe cooling methods and the right containers to make this happen. You can refrigerate the meals that you plan to eat within the next few days and then label and freeze all of the rest of them.

As we can see here, we are able to see a lot of benefits, and ease of use, when we are working with the idea of meal planning. It can be as simple or as complex as we would like. Some people spend a lot of o time working on meals and may get a whole month of meals up and running. And others are going to just work on a week at a time. You can customize this whole process to make it work for your needs, and it is particularly going to be useful for sticking with the vegan diet when you are ready to get started.

CHAPTER 3 - HOW TO GET YOUR KITCHEN READY

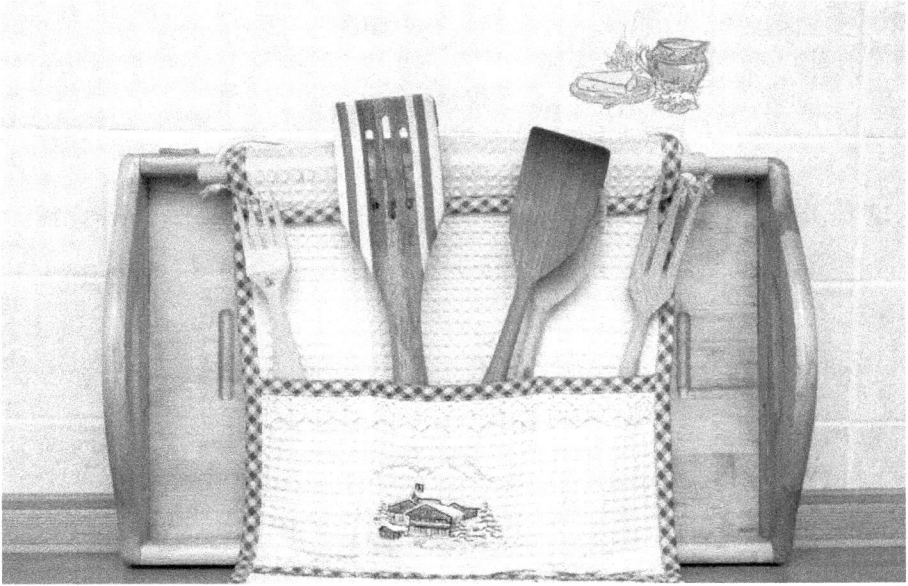

You will quickly find that working with the vegan diet is going to be a bit different than what you are able to see with the traditional diet that you may have been on up to this point. That is why we are going to spend a bit of time taking a look at how you can make sure that your kitchen is ready to go for this new change in your life.

As you can imagine, there are going to be a lot of great fruits and vegetables that you can add to your kitchen. Keeping your fridge full of these as much as possible is going to be a good step in the right direction when it is time to prepare yourself for this diet. Some good spices to get the food ready and lots of healthy whole grains and legumes can be a great way to get started.

With this in mind, and outside of some of the foods that you are naturally going to add into your kitchen when you choose this diet, we are going to take a look at some of the different appliances and tools that can be so useful when you go on this diet. You can choose whether you would like to add these into the kitchen and use them as a part of this diet plan or not. It all depends on the meals that you plan to create and what your overall goals are for this. Some of the tools and appliances that you are able to use when it is time to get your kitchen ready will include:

Spiralizer

While you are able to make some regular noodles and follow this diet plan, if you need to add in more fruits and vegetables to get your nutrients, you may find that working with a spiralizer in order to prepare your own plant-based noodles can be a great option to work with. You can do this with things like butternut squash or even zucchini noodles if you would like. There are a lot of these that you are able to go with at the grocery store.

A handheld spiralizer is not going to be that expensive to work with, but it is a bit more limited than other options. If you would like to be able to spiralize any kind of vegetable, then going with a countertop option is going to work well for this. They are a bit more in terms of cost, but they will come with a lot of the attachments that you need so that you are able to handle all of the noodles and more that you want to make in no time.

Cast Iron Skillet

The next option that we are going to be able to work with is a cast-iron skillet. If you take the time to treat this pan well, it is possible that you are going to have it forever. You will find that it is great for making the perfect pancakes and the expertly seared tofu as well. this is one of the essential tools for the home chef, whether they are working with the vegan diet or not. It is a non-stick pan without any commercial coatings that seem to be on some of the other pans that you can purchase well. You will also like they are oven safe and can be like a baking dish for some of your cobblers and more if you would like to work with this.

If you are going to get a cast-iron skillet, make sure that you learn some of the rules for breaking it in and how to take care of the skillet. This will ensure that you are getting the most out of it and that it is going to work for some of your cooking needs for a long time, even when you are focusing on the vegan diet.

Air Fryer

While this appliance may not be the most compact to work with, it is going to be really helpful when you are working with a vegan diet. You will find that you can quickly make room for it when you find out how easy it can make this kind of cooking on the vegan diet. Not only is it able to make light and crispy any food that you want, without any of the oil, this air-fryer is also going to help to cut down on the amount of time that you have to take cooking.

You can cook pretty much anything in your new air fryer, as long as you have taken care to find a good recipe to make this happen. It is good for frying tofu, working with some of the vegetables that can often give out some trouble, and more. It is so much better than the oven and can give you some of that fried food taste without all of the bad stuff in it.

Blender

The higher the quality that you can get with the blender, the better it is going to be for everyone. There are a lot of times when you will need to blend together lots of fruits and vegetables in this kind of diet, and taking the time to work with a high-quality blender is going to make a difference in how well that stuff turns out. There is a bit difference between the blenders out there, and if you really want to stick with the vegan diet, then you should go with one of the better ones, like Vitamix or Blendtec rather than saving money on one that is only $30.

This is a good investment when you are on this kind of diet plan and picking out one that is higher in quality and will last is going to be a good thing. This is often one that you are going to work with to help make some of your sweet treats, smoothies, and sauces along the way.

Along with the same idea, you may want to consider going with a food processor. Sometimes you can work with just one of the other depending on your own needs and what you are hoping to get out of this. Go with one that is going to be able to hold onto all of the foods that you need to make some of your meals. You don't want to go with one that is too big, but going with one that is a good size can make the difference in how much you are able to get done, especially if you are dealing with things like meal planning.

Steamer Basket

Another thing to consider is a steamer basket, especially one that is bamboo. You will find that unlike some of the steamer baskets that are usually offered with use in the microwave, this is going to be a great tool that will allow us to steam food in multiple layers. They are also going to be essential if you want to be able to cook some of your own buns or wantons that are homemade or if you want to work with creating some tamales.

If you are going to use one of these steamer baskets, make sure to line the bottom of this with some parchment paper. Cabbage leaves and a banana can work for this as well. having these in place will ensure that the food is not going to stick at all, and can help it to come out perfect each and every time.

As we can see, there are a number of tools that we are able to use to make cooking in the vegan diet so much easier than it would be in other situations. You can choose which option is the right one for you to use, and then leave out some of the ones that you don't think that you are going to want all that much. Sometimes, spending a few weeks working on meal planning and the vegan diet can give you a better idea of which items will be useful for you, and then you can go out and pick out the ones that you want, rather than wasting money on things and appliances that you will never use.

CHAPTER 4 - HEALTHY MEAL PLAN

Now it is time for us to get started on some of the basics that we are able to do in order to start on a weight loss meal prep program. If you want to see success with the vegan diet, one of the best things that you can do is sit down and work on meal prep. This is a harder diet to work with, and figuring out the meals at the last minute is not going to be as easy as we may like. We need to really think about what we want to make and have it all in front of us ahead of time. When we do this, we can figure out our macronutrients and the right amount of variety. And it is a whole lot easier.

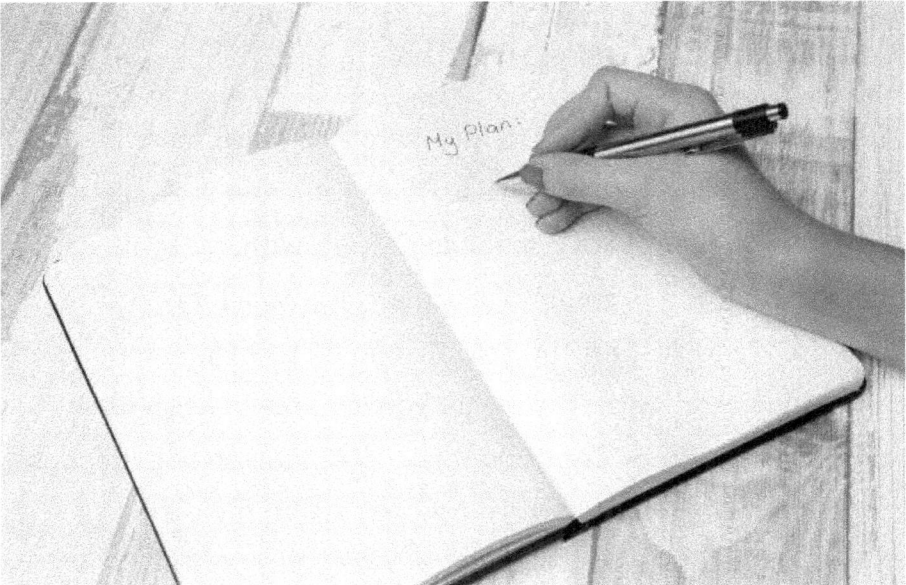

Think about it this way; when you are home from a long day at work and the kids are hungry and bouncing around, do you want to scramble around and hope that you are able to find the right ingredients to throw together a meal at the last minute? Or would it be better to just take something out of the fridge or the freezer, heat it up, and then dinner is done? And even better you will know that it fits on the vegan diet so you won't be questioning yourself along the way? This is possible when you work with your own meal prep program. Let's take a look now at a few of the steps that you can take in order to see more success with meal planning and how it can be a simple process to work with.

Learn About Your Diet Plan

The first step that we need to take here is to learn more about our diet plan that we want to use. The vegan diet is a very healthy meal plan that we are able to work with, and you will quickly see how it is going to provide you with a lot of health benefits. We took some time to talk about the vegan diet plan in this guidebook, but the more that you are able to learn about it, and the more you explore how this diet works and which foods are allowed and which ones you should avoid, the easier it is going to be to make it work.

There are a lot of parts that come with the vegan diet, and as you go through and try to make the right recipes and stick with this diet plan, you will find that a lot of questions will creep up. It is not uncommon to go through and look at a diet plan and wonder if one food or another will count for using it. Do some research and get a good understanding of what is allowed on the vegan diet so you can use it the right way.

Decide How Many Meals to Plan

This one is really going to depend on you and how much you want to get into all of this. Some people decide to just start with a few easy dinners to get the hang of it. Some want to plan out all of their meals and snacks each day of the week so they can grab and go without having to think about it. And some will try to do this for just a week, and others will do a few weeks or even a whole month so that they have some easy meals to put in the freezer and pull out when they need it.

You need to decide what is going to be the best for your own needs. This is going to let you know more about the different meals that you would like to create along the way. If you just want to do suppers, and you will just have oatmeal for breakfast, for example, then that may allow you to make some more meals at a time. Either way, knowing what meals you want to work with will ensure that you are set and will be able to pick out the right recipes for your needs.

Pick Out the Recipes You Want to Use

Once you know a bit more about the vegan diet and you have a good idea about which meals you need help with and how many you are going to prepare ahead of time, it is now time for you to go through and actually pick out which recipes you would like to add to your meal plan. Make sure to go with options that have a lot of variety in them. You do not want to get into the middle of your meal plan and start feeling bored with the foods that you get to consume.

There are a lot of different options that you are able to choose from when it comes to delicious vegan meals that are going to provide you with the nutrition and more that you are looking for. You will find that there are a lot of tasty options for meals to go within this guidebook, along with other books and even online with a simple search. Go ahead and save a bunch of them because it is easy to switch a few backs and forth as you make meal plans throughout the next few weeks.

Write Down Shopping List and Hit the Store

As you are going through all of the recipes that you want to create on this kind of diet plan, make sure that you write out the ingredients. You can get a sheet that separates these all out into different categories to make it easier, or just write them out as you go and organize them later. Make sure that you get all of the ingredients written down, and the right amounts, so that you do not have to guess later and you don't end up getting too much or too little.

Adding in some more organization to this process is going to make things a lot easier to handle. This will ensure that we are able to get some good results and save time at the grocery store. Once you are ready to head on over to the store, make sure that you stick to your list. Going off the list is not only going to cost you more at the store, but it is also going to make it more likely that you will pick up something that is unhealthy, whether it is part of the vegan diet or not. Stick with the list and you will always have exactly what you need when you work on this kind of diet plan.

Prepare the Ingredients

When you get home from the grocery store, it is time to prepare the ingredients. The way that you do this is going to depend on what kinds of foods you are trying to work with along the way. If you have a lot of produce, then go through and slice them all up and put into small containers or into little baggies so they are all together. If you are really organized and ready for the challenge, you can go through and separate them out based on how much is needed in the recipe. It is fine to go through and just add all of the same types into one container and sort them out later when making the recipes.

You may find that after grocery shopping, the idea of making all of these meals is going to be a challenge, and you may want to separate it out a little bit into two days. You can still go through and prepare the produce and other items so that when it is time to cook, whether it is that day or another day, you will have it all organized and ready to go for your own needs. Slice and dice now so that you can go right to the cooking later.

Make the Meals

Once you have gotten the recipes set up and all of the food prepared to go, this process should be easier. Always start with the things that will take the longest to make and work your way backward. This will ensure that you can keep moving and won't ever have to wait for something in the process. All of the cold meals that you are making, such as sandwiches or salads, should be done last so that you can prepare them while all of the other things are baking.

Keep some containers out as well, the ones that you plan to use in order to store some of the meals when they are done. Think about when you will use each of these and how long you plan to hold onto them before eating. If it is more than a few days, then put those meals into the freezer to keep them safe. The amount of time that this process is going to take really does depend on how many days of meals and how many meals a day that you would like to prepare. Start with just a week or a few meals to see what the process is about to make things easier.

Storing and Reheating

When the meals are all done and created, you will find that it is time to store them. The way that your store will depend on how far the process goes and how long you plan to use the meals. If you are only meal planning for a few days, you may be fine storing the foods in the fridge for that short amount of time. But if you want it to be available just on your busy nights or you don't plan to use it for a few weeks, then it is best to put it into the freezer.

When you are making the meal, try to determine how long you need to store it. If it is just a few days, putting it into a few Tupperware containers should be enough for your work. You can finish making the meals, or even just cutting up the fruits and vegetables, and then put them in the fridge, ready to grab and run off when you want.

On the other hand, if you are looking to store the food to have ready over the next week, or even the next month, then you will need to plan a bit more. Get some containers that are able to hold onto the meals and can be left in the freezer for some amount of time. You can then add the food to these containers, allow them to have some time to cool down after cooking, and then add them to the freezer. Make sure to add a label onto each of these. This will ensure that you are able to remember what is in each of the pans or containers when you take a look at them in the freezer.

The next part is where some of the planning is going to come into play. You will need to pull out some of the foods ahead of time to help them defrost if they have been put into the freezer. If you pull them out ten minutes before you need them, it is going to take a long time to get them nice and warm, and you will be frustrated. Knowing what you are going to eat each day of the week, and planning in that manner, is going to make things so much easier overall. You can pull out a few days' worth of food to defrost slowly in the fridge, and then they will be ready to heat up when the time comes.

Meal planning is a process that takes a bit of time, and it is not always as simple and easy as we may hope. It is not something that we are able to get done within just a few minutes, either. Instead, it is something that we need to really think about and plan out to get it all to fit together. But when we are able to do all of that, it will really make things easier on us overall and can ensure that we will see a lot more success when we go on this kind of diet plan.

PART 2

GETTING READY WITH THE MEAL PLAN

Chapter 5 - Your Weight Loss Meal Prep Program

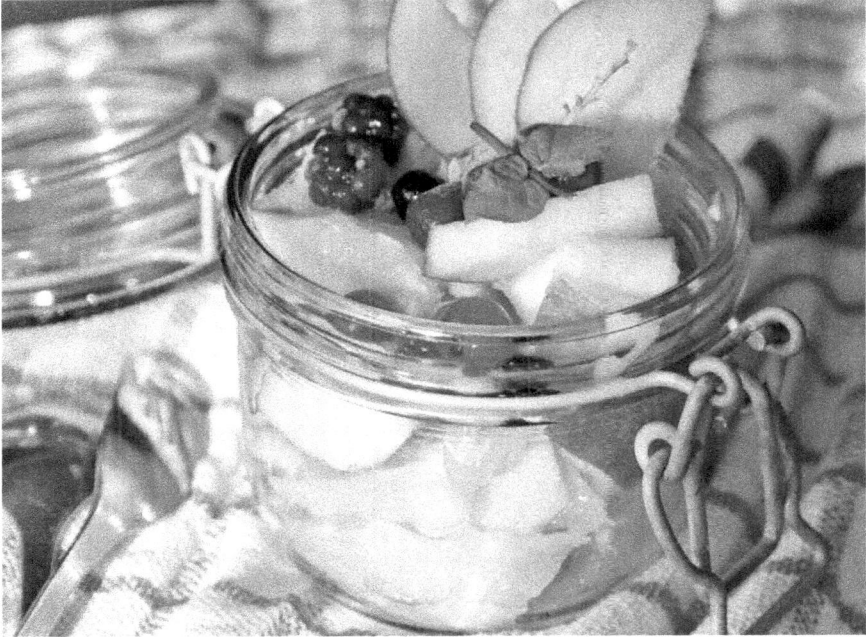

The next thing that we need to take a look at here is how we are able to use the idea of meal prepping and meal planning to help us to lose weight. Going on the vegan diet can be one of the best ways for you to lose weight and feel amazing, but you will also find that it is really hard to follow if you do not come up with a plan. If you are good at planning and think through some of your work ahead of time, you will find that it is a great diet plan. But without meal planning, you are going to spend too much time at home worrying about what to eat on for support or another meal way too often, and you will give up because you are too worn out and tired.

When it comes to eating healthy so that you can lose weight, failing to plan is the same as planning to fail. You can spend all day long exercising and doing all of the other things right, but if you are not consuming the right types of foods, or you are eating too much of the ones that are bad, you will find that all of the hard work in the world is not going to be shown off or on the scale.

Think about some of the thought and effort that you are able to put into your workouts. You think about what to wear, what workouts you are going to do, how intense and for how long, and what songs you want to add to the playlist. Doesn't it make sense that your nutrition should have a big impact on your weight as well and that you need to take some time to plan it out ahead of time as well?

Meal planning is going to be one of the main tools that you can use in order to achieve some of your own weight loss goals as well. Prepping your food ahead of time, whether that means that you are chopping up the fruits and vegetables that you want to use on a regular basis for the week, putting together some salads in a jar for the week, or doing extra batches of things and freezing them for later, you will find that meal planning is going to be one of the best options for your needs.

There are a lot of reasons that meal planning is going to be a good thing for you to try, especially when you are on the vegan diet and when you want to be able to lose a lot of weight quickly. Some of the different ways that meal planning can be good for you include the following:

1. It can save you from the takeout trap.

We have all been in this situation. We are tired, running low on time, and we are getting really hungry and angry at the same time. With all of these strikes going against you, you are going to be so much more vulnerable to the song of the fast-food or the pizza apps that can make life easier. After all, the whole idea of the convenience industry is designed to help cater to those who don't believe that they have the energy or the time to cook.

Meal planning is a nice option to go with because it is going to throw out all of those excuses ahead of time. When you have a lot of healthy meals that are prepped and all ready to go for you, some of the takeout options go from being a necessary evil to something that you do not need at all.

2. It can save a lot of time.

Spending a few hours during the week in the kitchen is not going to exactly top the list of our favorite ways to spend an afternoon. But you will find that it can help you to reap way more than a culinary reward from that one longer chunk of time than you would spending even half an hour cooking each evening during the week. It is possible to make a few weeks of meals in that sitting, and just have to throw it into the oven and have it ready throughout the whole week.

If you are a bit scared by the thought of trying to get all those meals done in one day then it is time to spend some time here doing smaller tasks. You could start out your meal prep with some of the tasks like marinating chicken breasts or chopping onions. This is going to work with making things easier, even if it doesn't do all of the things that you need later. That way, when you are going through a stressful day, you will not allow it to ruin your healthy intentions along the way.

3. Your snacks will be a lot smarter.

There are those days when we are all good and we start out on a positive path, patting ourselves on the back for eating a breakfast that is nutritious and a pretty good lunch. And then we get to the middle of the afternoon and that sugar craving is going to send us right to the vending machine or a cookie jar and that is not going to be good for our health.

We have to remember here that meal prep isn't going to always be the elaborate entrees. It is a chance to go through and plan some nutritious bites to have in between meals so we don't end up ruining our whole diet with the hunger cravings that we have during snack time. Creating a few options that you can keep on hand to help with all of this and to provide yourself with a vegan natural snack that will be so good for you.

4. It can take out the impulse buys.

When you are not on one of these meal plans, you will find that it is easier to add in unplanned and unnecessary additions to your grocery cart that will add to your budget and can make it really hard to stick with your weight loss goals. Creating a meal plan can then help to make a simple grocery list. You can make that list and only purchase the items that are on it, nothing else. This ensures that you just get healthy and nutritious meals, and nothing else.

5. Portion control is easier with this.

For those who are on a good weight loss journey, there is nothing better to focus on than portion control. When you are eating at a restaurant or using other methods to help you out, this can be hard. But meal prepping can make it so much easier to keep your portions under control. For weight management, you will find that portion sizes are going to be one of the most important things that you can follow. It helps you to make sure you are not taking on too many calories, fat, sodium, or more.

The typical American is taking on so much more than they need. Especially when we are eating out, the portion sizes have easily doubled or tripled through the years. If you do meal prepping and ensure that you do some good portion control, you are more in control over the amounts that you take in, which can do wonders for helping you to lose weight and cut out the calories effortlessly.

There are so many benefits that come with using the meal planning techniques when it comes to working on the vegan diet. When we are able to do it in the proper manner, you will find that the vegan diet is going to be easier to follow and can lead to a lot of natural and quick weight loss in the process.

Chapter 6 - Organizing Your Shopping List

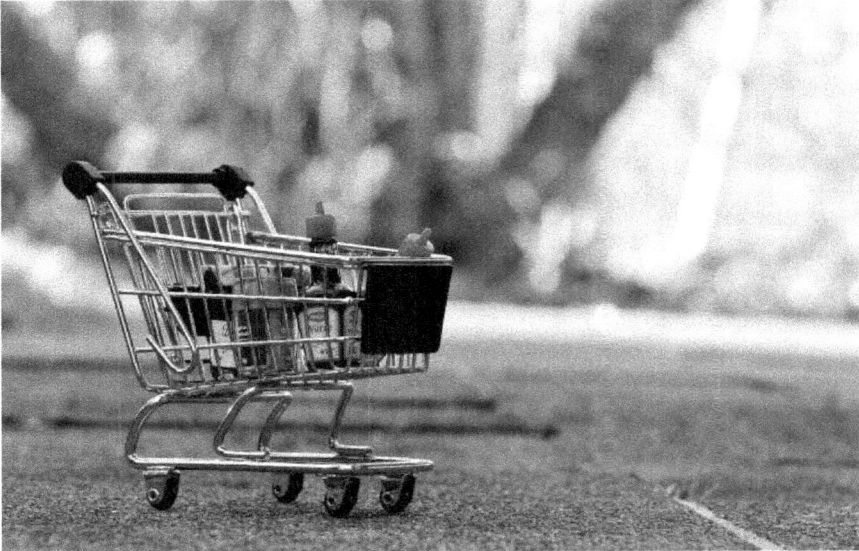

One of the things that we can do on this journey to make sure that we see the best results is to get some of our own grocery shopping lists all done. There are a lot of different ways that we can organize our list, but the more we think it out ahead of time, the more we can ensure that we will get into the store and out with all of the ingredients that we really need, and none of the ones that don't fit with our diet plan. It is also a good way to make sure that we can speed up the time it takes to be at the grocery store, and that is always good news.

The first thing that we need to do is make the shopping list. But it is kind of hard to make a shopping list without a good idea of the recipes that we need to use and want to rely on for the next week. Some people decide to go through the coupons and the store ads ahead of time and pick out a few recipes that look good based on the sales. If you are really into saving money and not wasting, then this is a good idea. If this is one of the first times that you have done any kind of meal planning, you may want to keep it a little bit easier and just pick out some of the recipes that sound good to you.

Remember that we are on the vegan diet plan, so pick out recipes that are going to fit with this. You can look through cookbooks, ask friends and family for some ideas, and even go online. There are a lot of great recipes, including the ones at the end of this guidebook, that you can use to help you get started. As you find the ones that you like, make sure to mark them in some manner so that you can remember where they are, and then go through and write it down on your calendar so you remember which day of your meal plan you would like to have it on.

As you are finding the recipes that you want to work with, make sure to write down the ingredients and how much of each you would like to work with. You can have these out of order for now. We are simply writing a few down to make sure that we have the necessary ingredients and that we don't forget anything. The organization doesn't have to be there right from the start because we can work on that later. Just get it all written down for the desired number of meals that you want.

When this part is done, you should have a nice list and all of the meals written down into your meal plan. Now it is time to get organized. You don't want to run back and forth to the bread aisle, for example, because you need a loaf of bread, some buns, and some tortilla shells but you wrote them down on different parts of the list so they were not right together. This is a hassle and can really cause some pains when you go to the grocery store.

If you can, try to go through and bring them into order in some manner. You can do this based on the aisle they are in based on your store, or even the food group they are in. you can have protein sources together, produce together, grains together and so on. Pick the method that is going to make the most sense for what you are doing at this time. You want the organization as much as possible.

If you are doing the online ordering, this can be even easier. Then you do not need to even organize the list at all. This can be a way to speed things up and saves you from spending that much time at the store at all. If this is offered in your area, it is something to give a try because it is going to make things a whole lot easier and saves you some time.

When you are in the store, make sure that you stick with the list that you made. Going off it can add in a lot of unhealthy items that you do not need at the store, and can make the cost go up. The vegan diet is sometimes a bit more expensive than some of the other diet plans that are out there, so having a method to keep the costs down, such as making a grocery list and sticking with it, can be one of the best ways to make this work for you.

And that is it. Making your own shopping list is not something that has to be very difficult and take up all of your time. You just need to have a plan and go through it one step at a time. When you are able to do this, it is a whole lot easier to see some good results in the process, and you will get in and out of the grocery store with all of the items that you need, and none of the ones that are just extras and won't help you stay on your goals.

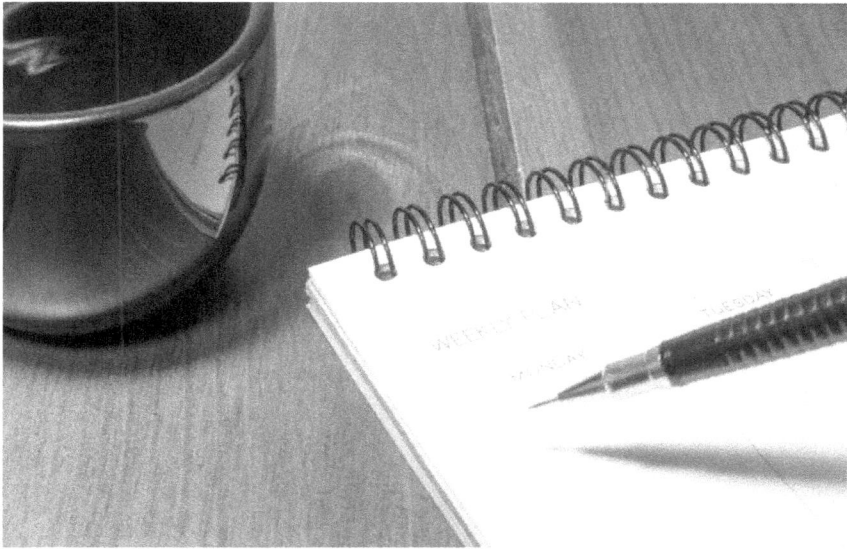

Week 1

Day 1:

Breakfast: Almond explosion

Snack: Hazelnut and chocolate bars

Lunch: Lentil, lemon and mushroom salad

Snack: Sunflower Protein Bars

Dinner: Black bean and quinoa burgers

Day 2:

Breakfast: Powerhouse protein shake
Snack: No-bake almond rice treats
Lunch: Sweet potato and black bean protein salad
Snack: overnight cookie dough oats
Dinner: Stuffed Indian Eggplant

Day 3:

Breakfast: Almond Protein Shake
Snack: matcha energy balls
Lunch: Southwest Style Salad
Snack: Lemon-lime pie bars
Dinner: Sweet potato sushi

Day 4:

Breakfast: Cranberry Protein Shake
Snack: mocha chocolate brownie bars
Lunch: Cuban Tempeh Buddha Bowl
Snack: Nutty blueberry snack bars
Dinner Tofu Cacciatore

Day 5:

Breakfast: Avocado Protein Shake
Snack: Cranberry vanilla protein bars
Lunch: Shaved Brussel Sprouts Salad
Snack: Spicy Chickpea poppers
Dinner: High Protein Black Bean Dip

Shopping List for Week 1:

1. 1 package brown rice syrup
2. 1 package cashew butter
3. 1 package cocoa powder
4. 1 package of hazelnuts
5. 1 package of chocolate-flavored protein powder
6. 1 package of vanilla vegan protein powder
7. 1 package of peanut butter
8. 1 package of almonds
9. 1 package of raisins
10. 1 package of oatmeal
11. 2 packages of almond milk, unsweetened
12. 1 package of nutmeg
13. 1 package of cinnamon
14. 1 package of vanilla
15. 1 package of sunflower butter
16. 1 bottle of maple syrup

17. 1 package of puffy rice cereal

18. 2 packages of oats

19. 1 package arugula

20. 1 package cilantro

21. 1 lemon

22. 1 package chili flakes

23. 1 package garlic powder

24. 1 bottle olive oil

25. 9 purpose or sweet onions

26. 1 package mushrooms

27. 1 package lentils

28. 1 package spirulina

29. 1 package kale

30. 1 package spinach

31. 1 pineapple

32. 2 green apples

33. 1 package of lettuce

34. 1 package of pepper

35. 1 package of paprika powder

36. 1 package red pepper lakes

37. 1 package of flour, whole wheat

38. 1 garlic head

39. 2 green and 2 red bell peppers

40. 1 package of quinoa

41. 3 packages of black beans

42. 1 package salt

43. 1 package of onion powder

44. 2 cans chickpeas

45. 1 package dried cranberries

46. 1 package walnuts

47. 1 package slivered almonds

48. 1 package Brussels sprouts

49. 1 package balsamic vinegar

50. 28 ounces of diced tomatoes

51. 1 package carrots

52. 1 package dried blueberries

53. 14 oz. tempeh

54. 1 package basmati rice

55. 1 package coffee, brewed

56. 1 bottle of coconut milk

57. 1 package hemp seeds

58. 1 banana

59. 1 package cranberries

60. 1 package tamari

61. 1 package agave nectar

62. 1 package rice vinegar

63. 1 package nori sheets

64. 2 packages of silken tofu

65. 1 package of sunflower seeds

66. 1 package pecans

67. 1 package chia seeds

68. 1 bottle of vinegar

69. 1 package chili powder

70. 1 package corn

71. 3 avocados

72. 7 cherry tomatoes

73. 1 package of mixed greens

74. 1 package garbanzo beans

75. 1 package matcha powder

76. 1 package dates

77. 1 package pistachios

78. 1 package cashews, raw

79. 1 package coconut milk

80. 1 bottle of soymilk

81. 1 package turmeric

82. 1 package cumin

83. 1 package coconut sugar

84. 2 packages tomato paste

85. 3 Roma tomatoes

86. 6 eggplants

87. 1 package flaxseed

88. 1 package parsley

89. 1 package cayenne

90. 1 sweet potato

91. 1 package, coconut shredded

92. 1 package almond butter

93. 1 package protein powder, no flavor

94. 1 bottle of coconut water.

Week 2

Day 1:

Breakfast: Banana protein punch
Snack: Chocolate and zucchini muffins
Lunch: Colorful protein salad
Snack: Energy Crackers
Dinner: Mango-Tempeh Wraps

Day 2:

Breakfast: Almond protein shake
Snack: sunflower protein bars
Lunch: Creamy squash pizza
Snack: chewy almond butter balls
Dinner: Edamame and Ginger Salad

Day 3:

Breakfast: Cranberry Protein Shake
Snack: Overnight Cookie Dough Oats
Lunch: Super Summer Salad
Dinner: Nutty Blueberry Snack Squares
Dinner: Sweet potato chili

Day 4:

Breakfast: Avocado Protein Shake
Snack: Peanut butter and banana cookies
Lunch: Vegan Mushroom pho
Snack: Almond and date bars.
Diner: Ruby Red Beet Burgers

Day 5:

Breakfast: Almond and date protein bars
Snack: Tropical protein smoothie
Lunch: Lasagna fungo
Snack: Savory sweet lentil bites
Dinner Portobello burgers

Shopping List for Week 2:

1. 1 package onion flakes
2. 1 package chia seeds
3. 1 package flax seeds
4. 1 lemon
5. 10 carrots
6. 1 package kale

7. 1 package of cabbage, green or purp_e

8. 1 head of garlic

9. 1 package green onions

10. 1 package navy beans

11. 1 package vanilla

12. 1 thing of nutmeg

13. 1 thing of cinnamon

14. 1 thing baking powder

15. 1 bottle or carton of almond milk

16. 1 package of chocolate chips, vegan

17. 1 zucchini

18. 1 package of maple syrup

19. 1 jar of applesauce

20. 7 bananas

21. 1 thing olive oil

22. 1 thing of coconut oil

23. 1 thing of pepper

24. 2 quinoa packages

25. 1 thing salt

26. 1 bottle or carton of oat milk

27. 3 things of almonds

28. 1 package chocolate protein powder

29. 1 package vanilla protein powder

30. 1 thing of chili powder

31. 2 buns or wraps

32. 1 thing of mushrooms, portobello

33. 1 thing of sunflower seeds

34. 1 thing of allspice

35. 1 thing of nutritional yeast

36. 1 thing of hummus

37. 1 thing of lasagna noodles

38. 1 thing of hemp seeds

39. 1 carton of blueberries

40. 1 orang

41. 1 thing of parsley

42. 1 thing of balsamic vinegar

43. 1 thing of garbanzo beans

44. 2 beets

45. 1 package cranberries, dried

46. 1 thing bean sprouts, raw

47. 1 package of rice noodles

48. 1 thing of hoisin sauce

49. 1 thing of mushrooms

50. 1 thing cocoa nibs

51. 1 carton coconut milk

52. 1 thing cacao powder

53. 4 packages of tofu

54. 2 sweet potatoes

55. 1 can diced tomatoes with green chilis

56. 1 thing of sweet onions

57. 1 package of dried blueberries

58. 1 package chickpeas

59. 1 thing of radishes

60. 1 bushel of Brussels sprouts

61. 1 thing of beans, red kidney

62. 1 package of basil

63. 1 package of rolled oats

64. 1 lime

65. 1 carton of orange juice

66. 1 bottle sesame oil

67. 1 package of ginger

68. 2 packages of green lentils

69. 1 thing of edamame

70. 1 thing of mint

71. 3 avocados

72. 1 package puffy rice cereal

73. 1 package of vanilla

74. 1 jar of almond butter

75. 1 thing of carb chips

76. 1 thing of onion powder

77. 1 onion, purple

78. 1 thing of French lentils

79. 1 head of broccoli

80. 1 red and one green bell pepper

81. 1 thing of paprika

82. 1 thing of cumin

83. 1 thing of oregano

84. Red pepper flakes

85. 2 squash, butternut
86. Cocoa powder
87. 1 carton of milk, soy
88. 1 thing of garlic powder
89. 1 lettuce head
90. 3 mangoes
91. 1 package sweet chili sauce
92. 2 tempeh packages
93. Paprika powder
94. 1 thing of sesame seeds
95. 2 things of cashews
96. 2 things of pumpkin seeds
97. 2 things of peanuts

Week 3

Day 1:

Breakfast: cinnamon and apple protein smoothie
Snack: Lemon-lime pie bars
Lunch: Portobello burritos
Snack: Lentil radish salad
Dinner: Mushroom madness stroganoff

Day 2:

Breakfast: Candied protein trail mix
Snack: Cake batter smoothie
Lunch: Creamy squash pizza
Snack: Chocolate and zucchini muffins
Dinner: Sweet and Sour Tofu

Day 3:

Breakfast; Chewy Almond butter balls
Snack: Energy Crackers
Lunch: Moroccan eggplant stew
Snack: Mocha chocolate brownie bars
Dinner: Taco Tempeh Salad

Day 4:

Breakfast: Banana Protein Punch
Snack: Sunflower Protein Bars
Lunch: Ratatouille
Snack: Spicy chickpea poppers
Dinner: BBQ Greens and Grits

Day 5:

Breakfast: Avocado Chia Protein Shake
Snack: Cranberry Vanilla Protein Bars
Lunch: Roasted Almond Protein Salad
Snack: Lemon Lime Pie Bars
Dinner: Sweet Potato Quesadillas

Shopping List for Week 3

1. Cherry tomatoes, 3
2. Radishes, 2
3. Silken tofu, 1 package
4. Brown lentils, 1 package
5. Chickpeas, 1 package
6. Sesame oil, 1 container
7. Miso paste, 1 package

8. Maple syrup, 1 bottle

9. Flour, 1 package

10. Jalapeno, 1

11. Red onion, 1

12. Tomatoes, 1 container

13. Cilantro, 1 bunch

14. Avocados, 3

15. Potatoes, 2

16. Portobello mushrooms, 1 package

17. Lemons, 2

18. Dates, 1 package

19. Raw cashews, 2 packages

20. Pecans, 2 containers

21. Chia seeds, 2 containers

22. Coconut oil, 1 container

23. Olive oil, 1 bottle

24. Chocolate protein powder, 1 package

25. Vanilla protein powder, 1 package

26. Pepper

27. Salt

28. Cinnamon, 1 container

29. Coconut milk, 2 cartons

30. Green apple, 1

31. Garlic powder

32. Chickpeas, 2 cans

33. Basil, 1 bunch

34. Yellow squash, 1
35. Fennel seeds, 1 package
36. Heirloom tomatoes, 2
37. Sunflower butter, 1 container
38. Oat milk, 1 carton
39. Kale, 1 bunch
40. Lime, 1
41. Jalapeno, 1
42. Tempeh, 2 packages
43. Black beans, 1 package
44. Brewed coffee, 1 package
45. Agave nectar, 1 package
46. Cocoa powder, 1 package
47. Sweet onions, 1 package
48. Tomato sauce, 1 package
49. Green lentils, 1 package
50. Allspice, 1 package
51. Eggplants, 2
52. Turmeric, 1 package
53. Golden raisins, 1 package
54. Garbanzo beans, 1 package
55. Peanuts, 1 package
56. Onion flakes
57. Flaxseeds, 1 container
58. Almond butter, 1 jar
59. Puffy rice cereal, 1 package

60. Carob chips, 1 package

61. Coconut sugar, 1 package

62. Cornstarch, 1 package

63. Drained tofu, 2 packages

64. Soy sauce, 1 package

65. Rice vinegar, 1 bottle

66. Bell pepper, red, 1

67. Green bell peppers, 2

68. White onions, 2

69. Ginger root, 1

70. Pineapple, 1

71. Quinoa, 2 packages

72. Zucchini, 2

73. Baking powder, 1

74. Applesauce, 1 jar

75. Purple onions, 2

76. Red pepper flakes, 1 package

77. Oregano, 1 package

78. Paprika, 1 package

79. Cumin, 1 package

80. Onion powder, 1 package

81. Garlic, 1 head

82. French green lentils, 1 package

83. Broccoli, 1 head

84. Butternut squash, 2

85. Almond milk, 2 cartons

86. Vanilla, 1
87. Oats, 2 packages
88. Cashew butter, 1 jar
89. Bananas, 5
90. Nutmeg, 1
91. Walnuts, 2 containers
92. Almonds, 3 containers
93. Apple cider vinegar, 1 bottle
94. Spinach, 2 packages
95. Thyme
96. Mushrooms, 1 package
97. Tomato paste, 1 package
98. Tamari sauce, 1 package
99. Almond flour, 1 package
100. Noodles, 1 package
101. Sesame seeds, 1 package.
102. Sweet potato, 1
103. Rice, 1 package
104. Navy beans, 1
105. Dried cranberries, 1
106. The coconut that is shredded, 1
107. Peanut butter, 1 jar
108. Smoked paprika, 1
109. Grits, 1
110. Collard greens, 1
111. Cayenne, 1

Week 4

Day 1:

Breakfast: Cinnamon and apple protein smoothie
Snack Nutty, blueberry snack squares.
Lunch: Stuffed Eggplant
Dinner: Savory Sweet Lentil Bites
Dinner: Teriyaki Tofu Wraps

Day 2:

Breakfast: Mocha Chocolate Brownie Bars
Snack: Cookie Dough Oats
Lunch: Satay Tempeh
Snack: Banana Protein Punch
Dinner: Tex-Mex Tofu and Beans

Day 3:

Breakfast: Almond Explosion
Snack: Matcha Energy Balls
Lunch: Stuffed Sweet Potatoes
Snack: Sunflower Protein Bars
Dinner: Red Beans and Rice

Day 4:

Breakfast; Cranberry Protein Shake

Snack: Hazelnut and Chocolate Protein Bars

Lunch: Coconut Tofu Curry

Snack Almond and date protein bars

Dinner: Tahini Falafels

Day 5:

Breakfast: Almond Protein Shake

Snack: Energy Crackers

Lunch: Black Bean Dip

Snack: Lemon Lime Pie Bars

Dinner: Baked Enchilada Bowls

Shopping List for Week 4

1. White onion, 1
2. Almond butter, 1 jar
3. Shredded coconut, 1 package
4. Sunflower seeds, 1 package
5. Allspice, 1 package
6. Coconut oil, 1 container
7. Green lentils,1 package

8. Green bell peppers,5

9. Turmeric, 1 thing

10. Cumin, 1 thing

11. Coconut sugar, 1 package

12. Tomato paste, 1 can

13. Garlic, 1 head

14. Spinach, 1 package

15. Olive oil, 1 container

16. Purple onions, 3

17. Roma tomatoes, 3

18. Eggplants, 6

19. Black beans, 3 packages

20. Pepper

21. Salt

22. Dried blueberries, 1 package

23. Maple syrup, 1 bottle

24. Puffy rice cereals, 1 package

25. Cashews, 4 packages with 2 raw

26. Almonds, 2 packages with 1 raw

27. Green apple, 1

28. Chocolate protein powder, 1 package

29. Vanilla protein powder,1 package

30. Cinnamon, 1 thing

31. Coconut milk, 1 carton

32. Nutritional yeast, 1

33. Apple vinegar, 1 bottle

34. Flour, 1 package
35. Oregano, 1
36. MCT oil, 1 bottle
37. Sweet potato,1
38. Pecans, 1 container
39. Onion powder, 1 thing
40. Pumpkinseeds, 1 package
41. Onion flakes, 1
42. Soymilk, 1 carton
43. Broccoli,1 head
44. Tahini, 1 package
45. Chickpeas, 1 package
46. Dried cranberries, 1 package
47. Applesauce, 1 jar
48. Tomatoes, 2
49. Coconut milk, 1 can
50. Peas, 1 package
51. Turmeric,1 package
52. Cashew butter, 1 jar
53. Curry powder 1 thing
54. Brown rice syrup, 1 bottle
55. Hemp seeds, 1 package
56. Chia seeds, 1 package
57. Cranberries, 1
58. Celery ribs, 1
59. Parsley flakes, 1

60. Basil, 1
61. Cauliflower, 1
62. Red beans, 1
63. Sunflower butter, 1 jar
64. Pistachios, 1 package
65. Matcha powder, 1
66. Hazelnuts, 1
67. Dates, 1
68. Raisins, 1
69. Lemons, 2
70. Chili powder, 1
71. Avocado, 1
72. Paprika, 1
73. Tofu, 1
74. Brown rice, 1
75. Banana, 3
76. Oat milk, 1 carton
77. Purple cabbage, 1
78. Cauliflower rice, 1
79. Tempeh, 2
80. Red pepper flakes, 1
81. Rice vinegar, 1 bottle
82. Ginger root, 1
83. Peanut butter, 1 jar
84. Flaxseeds, 1
85. Almond milk, 2 cartons

86. Agave nectar, 1 package
87. Brewed coffee, 1 package
88. Vanilla, 1
89. Nutmeg
90. Oats, 2
91. Pineapple, 1
92. Sesame seeds, 1
93. Lettuce, 1 package
94. Sesame oil, 1 bottle,
95. Soy sauce, 1 bottle.

PART 3

THE RECIPES

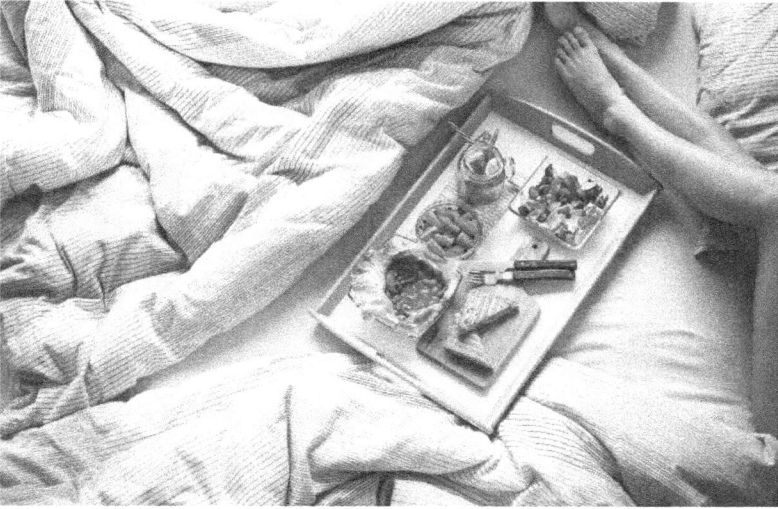

Cinnamon and Apple Protein Smoothie

What's inside:

Matcha powder, 2 tsp.)

Ice cubes (3)

Cinnamon (.5 tsp.)

Coconut milk (1 c.)

Vegan protein powder, vanilla (2 scoops)

Apple, green ad chopped (1)

How to make this:

1. Take out your blender and add all of the ingredients above inside. Let these blend together for about 2 minutes.
2. When this is done move the shake to a big cup or to a shaker. Top it all with some of the cinnamon powder and enjoy.

**

Tropical Protein Smoothie

What's inside:

Ice cubes (6)

Guarana (1 tsp.)

Hemp seeds (1 Tbsp.)

Vegan protein powder, choose chocolate or vanilla (2 scoops)

blueberries (.5 c.)

Mango chunks (1 c)

Peeled and parted orange (1)

How to make this

1. To start this recipe, bring out your blender and add in all of your ingredients, along with the guarana.
2. Put the lid on top and then let this mix for a few minutes. After two minutes, you can transfer the shake to a shaker or a cup and enjoy it.

***

Cranberry Protein Shake

What's inside:

Ice cubes (4)

Coconut milk (2 c.)

Hemp seeds (.25 c.)

Chia seeds (.25 c.)

Banana (1)

Vegan protein powder, vanilla or chocolate (2 scoops)

Cranberries (.25 c.)

How to make this:

1. Go through and soak the chia seeds for a few hours before starting this recipe.
2. When the chia seeds are done with the soaking, you can add them along with the rest of the ingredients into your blender.
3. Add the lid on top of the blender and then blend all of these together for a few minutes.
4. When this is done, move the mixture to some large cups and serve.

***

Strawberry and Orange Smoothie

What's inside:

Ice cubes (2)

Vanilla vegan protein powder (3 scoops)

Banana (1)

Orange (1)

Strawberries (10)

Coconut milk (2 c.)

How to make this

1. To start this recipe, bring out a blender and add in all of the ingredients that we are using.
2. Add the lid on top of the blender and let the ingredients mix together for a few minutes.
3. When the two minutes are up, move this over to a big cup and then serve.

***

Powerhouse Protein Shake

What's inside:

Unflavored protein powder (2 scoops)

Coconut water (1 c.)

Spirulina (1 tsp)

Drained and rinsed spinach (1 c.)

Chopped kale (1 c.)

Pineapple chunks (1 c.)

Chopped green apple (2)

How to make this:

1. Take all of the ingredients and add them to your prepared blender.
2. Put the lid on top of the blender and then let these mix together for about 2 minutes.
3. After that is done, move to a large cup and ten enjoy.

***

Avocado Protein Shake

What's inside:

Cacao powder (2 tsp.)

Ice cubes (3)

Water (1 c.)

Chocolate protein powder (2 scoops)

Peanut butter (1.5 Tbsp.)

Pitted and peeled avocado (.5)

Coconut milk (1 c.)

Dry chia seeds (.25 c.)

How to make this:

1. Take a bit of time before making this to soak the chia seeds. After a few hours, you can drain out the water that is left.
2. Add in these chia seeds and any of the other ingredients to your blender. Blend these together for a few minutes to make smooth.
3. Move the shake to a bit cup and then add a bit of cacao powder on top before serving.

Almond Protein Shake

What's inside:

Cacao powder (1 tsp.)

Ice cubes (4)

Chocolate protein powder (2 scoops)

Coconut oil (1 Tbsp.)

Maple syrup (1 tsp.)

Almonds (3 Tbsp)

Soymilk (1.5 c.)

How to make this:

1. Bring out your blender and then add all of the ingredients inside.
2. Blend all of the ingredients together for a few minutes. And when this is done, add the shake to a large shaker or cup and then serve.

***

Oatmeal Protein Mix

What's inside:

Peanut butter (2 Tbsp.)
Ice cubes (2)
Almond milk (1 c.)
Almonds (.25 c.)
Maple syrup (.5 tsp.)
Cinnamon (.5 tsp.)
Chocolate vegan protein powder (3 scoops)
Oatmeal, dry (1 c.)

How to make this

1. Bring out your blender and add in all of the ingredients that are listed above.
2. When this is ready, add the lid to the top of the blender and mix the ingredients together for two minutes.
3. When that is done, move to a big cup or to your shaker before enjoying it.

Almond Explosion

What's inside:

Ice cubes (2)

Cinnamon (.5 tsp.)

Vanilla protein powder (3 scoops)

Peanut butter (3 Tbsp.)

Water (.5 c.)

Almonds (.5 c.)

Raisins (.5 c.)

Dry oatmeal (.5 c.)

Almond milk (1.5 c.)

How to make this:

1. Take out your blender and get it all set up. When ready, you can add in all of the ingredients to the blender.
2. Add the lid on top of the blender. Allow this to blend together for a few minutes.
3. After this time, transfer to a large cup. Add some ice cubes if you want to keep this cool or microwave for a nice treat.

***

Banana Protein Punch

What's inside:

Maple syrup (1 Tbsp.)

Vegan protein powder, vanilla or chocolate (2 scoops)

Water (.5 c.)

Almonds (.5 c.)

Almond milk (1 c.)

Bananas (2)

How to make this:

1. Take out the blender and get it all set up. Add in all of the ingredients above to your blender and then blend them together for a few minutes.
2. Pour this into a large cup or your shaker and then enjoy it.

***

Pecan and Maple Granola

What's inside:

Ground cinnamon (.5 tsp.)
Maple syrup (.25 c)
Vanilla (1 tsp.)
Pecan pieces (.25 c.)
Rolled oats (1.5 c.)

How to make this:

1. Turn on the oven to start this and give it time to heat up to 300 degrees. While the oven is heating up, take out a baking sheet and line it with some parchment paper.
2. Then, take out a big bowl and combine together the cinnamon, vanilla, maple syrup, pecan pieces, and the oats. Stir these until the pecan pieces and the oats are coated all the way through.
3. When those are combined, you can spread this mixture out onto the baking sheet that you prepared ad then make it into an even layer. Add to the oven to bake.
4. After about 20 minutes, with a check on them at ten minutes, the granola should be all done. Take these out of the oven and let them set on the counter to cool down for a bit before serving.

Overnight Oatmeal

What's inside:

Chia seeds (1 Tbsp.)
Maple syrup (1 Tbsp.)
Sliced banana (1)
Pineapple chunks (.5 c.)
Diced mango (.5 c.)
Milk that is plant-based (2 c.)
Rolled oats (2 c.)

How to make:

1. Bring out a big bowl and mix together the chia seeds, maple syrup, banana, pineapple, mango, milk, and oats.
2. When this is done, cover up the bowl and add it to the fridge. This needs to set for at least four hours, though leaving it to sit overnight is usually going to be the best.
3. The next morning you can take this out and serve.

***

Pumpkin Pie Oatmeal

What's inside:

Ground nutmeg (.25 tsp.)
Ground cloves (.25 tsp.)
Ground cinnamon (1 tsp.)
Maple syrup (2 Tbsp.)
Unsweetened pumpkin puree (1 c.)
Oats (1 c.)
Milk that is plant-based (3 c.)

How to make this:

1. Brin gout a pan and heat it up on medium heat. Add the milk inside and then let this come to a boil.
2. When the milk is to a rolling boil, you can reduce the heat down to a low and then stir in the nutmeg, cloves, cinnamon, maple syrup, oats, and pumpkin puree.
3. When all of those are in the pot, cover it up and let these cook for a bit. You will want to stop and stir it every few minutes to help keep it mixed and to make sure that none of the oatmeal is able to stick to the bottom.
4. After about half an hour, this mixture should be done. Pour it into a few bowls before serving.

Peanut Butter and Chocolate Quinoa

What's inside:

Peanut powder (1 Tbsp.)

Cocoa powder (1 Tbsp.)

Maple syrup (1 Tbsp.)

Cooked quinoa (2 c.)

Milk that is based on plants (1 c.)

1. Take the time to cook up the quinoa. You can follow the instructions that are on the back of the box that came with it to make this easier.
2. When that is done, bring out another pan and heat it up. Add the milk inside and bring this to a boil as well.
3. When the milk is at a rolling boil, then it is time to reduce the heat a bit to a low setting before adding in the peanut powder, cocoa powder, maple syrup, and the quinoa.
4. Cook these for a bit without the lid on top. After five minutes, with a constant stream of stirring the whole time, you can serve this mixture nice and warm.

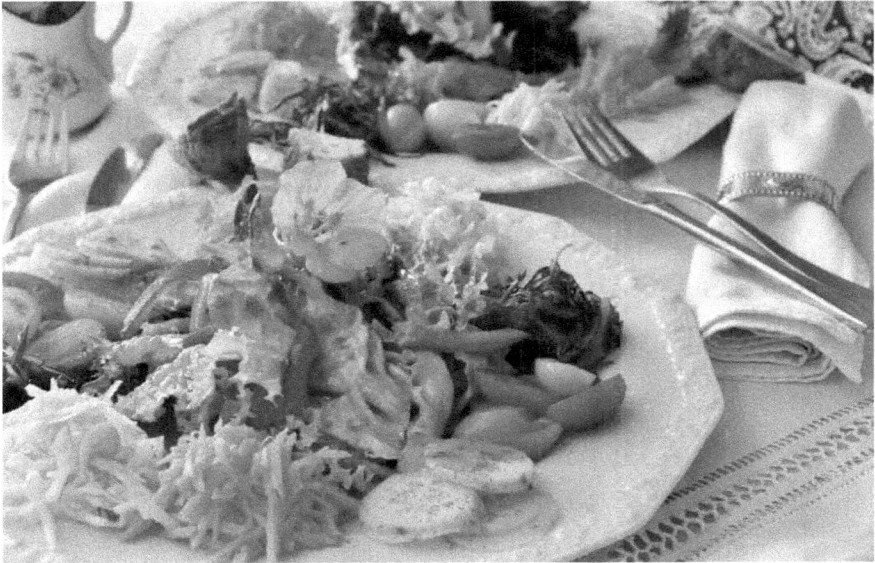

Lentil and Mushroom Salad

What's inside:

Pepper

Salt

Arugula (.5 c.)

Chopped cilantro (2 Tbsp.)

Lemon juice (1 Tbsp.)

Chili flakes (.25 tsp.)

Garlic powder (2 Tbsp.)

Olive oil (4 tsp.)

Chopped purple onion (1 c.)

Sliced mushrooms (3 c.)

Vegetable broth (2 c.)

Dry lentils (.5 c.)

How to make this:

1. Take some time to sprout the lentils using the method of your choice. When that is done, take the vegetable stock and bring it to a boil in a pan on your stove.
2. Add the lentils to this boiling broth and then cover up the pan. Let these cook until the lentils start to get a bit tender.
3. After 5 minutes, you can take the pan off the heat and then drain the extra water.
4. Then add in a frying pan over high heat and then add in two tablespoons of olive oil. When that is warm, add in the chili flakes, garlic, and onions.
5. Cook this one until the onions start to turn translucent, which can take around ten minutes. Add the mushrooms to this and mix around well.
6. Continue to cook for a bit until the onions and mushrooms are done. Take the pan from the heat.
7. Mix the garlic, mushrooms, onions, and lentils in a big bowl. Add the lemon juice and then top with the rest of the oil. Toss or stir to make sure that it is combined well.
8. Serve this mixture over the arugula in a bowl, adding some of the pepper and salt to taste as you would like.

Sweet Potato and Black Bean Salad

What's inside:

Pepper

Salt

Parsley (.25 c.)

Cayenne (.25 tsp.)

Chili powder (.5 Tbsp.)

Minced garlic (1 Tbsp.)

Lime juice (2 Tbsp.)

Olive oil (2 Tbsp.)

Chopped purple onion (1 c.)

Sweet potato (1)

Spinach (4 c.)

Dry black beans (1 c.)

How to make this

1. Take some time to preheat the black beans. Turn on the oven and let it heat up to 400 degrees.
2. Slice up the sweet potatoes into little cubes and then add to a bowl. Then add in the salt, olive oil, and onions.
3. Toss these ingredients around until the onions and sweet potatoes are completely coated and then add to a baking

sheet that has been lined with some parchment paper. Make sure to spread them out in a single layer.

4. Add these to the oven and let them cook for a bit until the sweet potatoes start to become crispy and brown.

5. After 40 minutes, the potatoes and the rest of the mixture will be done. In the meantime, you can take out a bowl and combine the cayenne, chili powder, garlic, lime juice, and the rest of the olive oil.

6. When the potatoes are done, take them out of the oven and move them to the big bowl. Then top with the salt, parsley, and black beans. Toss these around to combine well.

7. Mix in the spinach and then serve.

***

Super Summer Salad

What's inside:

For the dressing
Avocado, diced (1)
Water (.25 c.)
Salt
Chopped basil (.25 c.)
Lemon juice (1 tsp.)
Olive oil (1 Tbsp.)
For the salad
Pepper
Salt
Dry chickpeas (.25 c.)
Flaxseeds (1 tsp.)
Red kidney beans (.25 c.)
Sliced radishes (2)
Chopped walnuts (1 Tbsp.)
Brussel sprouts (2 c.)
Shredded kale (4 c.)

How to make this:

1. We can go through this and prepare the kidney beans and the chickpeas according to the method we like the moat.
2. Take out a small bowl and soak up the flax seeds for a few minutes or more. When that time is done, drain out the extra water.
3. Now it is time to prepare the dressing. To do this, bring out a blender and add in all the ingredients for the dressing including half the avocado, lemon juice, salt, olive oil, and basil.
4. Pulse this at a low speed and add in some smaller amounts of water until the dressing is smooth and creamy and then add to a bowl and set to the side.
5. Now it is time to bring out a big bowl and mix together the rest of the avocado with the walnuts, radishes, kidney beans, kale, Brussel sprouts, kale, and chickpeas.
6. Serve this with the dressing and the flax seeds on top.

***

Roasted Almond Protein Salad

What's inside:

Chopped purple onion (.25 c.)

Spinach (4 c.)

Dry quinoa (.5 c.)

Navy beans, dry (.5 c.)

Dash of chili powder

Cayenne (.5 tsp.)

Paprika (.5 tsp.)

Chickpeas dry (.5 c.)

Salt

Olive oil (1 tsp.)

Whole almonds, raw (.5 c.)

How to make this:

1. Take out a pan and add the water and quinoa to it. Cook the quinoa-based on the instructions cn the box and then store it in the fridge when it is done.
2. Then you can go through the process of preparing the beans as well. when those are done add to the fridge as well.

3. Bring out a bowl and stir together the olive oil, salt, spices, and almonds and stir to make them nice and coated.

4. Take out a skillet and heat it up. When it is nice and warm, add the almond mixture to this. You can roast this while stirring the almonds around so that they can get browned all over. You may hear that it is going to crackle and pop a bit in the skillet and that is normal for this one.

5. After 5 minutes, making sure to stir around the whole time to prevent burning, you can turn off the heat and toss in the onions, cooked quinoa, beans, spinach, and more to the skillet. Stir it well before moving to a bowl.

6. Enjoy this salad with some of the dressing of your choice.

***

Lentil Radish Salad

What's inside:

Dressing
Pepper
Salt
Miso paste, white (1 Tbsp.)
Sesame oil (.5 Tbsp.)
Olive oil (1 Tbsp.)
Maple syrup (1 Tbsp.)

Water (1 Tbsp.)

Lemon juice (1 Tbsp.)

For the salad

Dry chickpeas (.5 c.)

Brown lentils, dry (.25 c.)

Silken tofu (14 oz.)

Roasted sesame seeds (.25 c.)

Halved cherry tomatoes (.5 c.)

Mixed greens (5 c.)

Sliced radishes (2)

How to make this:

1. Take the time to prepare both the lentils and the chickpeas with the help of a favorite method.
2. When that is done, add all of the ingredients that we are using for the dressing into the food processor or blender. Mix this on a low setting until it is nice and smooth, adding in the water necessary to get it to the right consistency of your choice.
3. Add some pepper and salt to taste and a bit more water to this to make it just right before setting to the side.
4. Now it is time to cut the tofu into some smaller cubes. Then you can add this to a bowl with the tomatoes, radishes, chickpeas, mixed greens, and lentils.
5. Add in the dressing and then mix it all together. Top with some roasted sesame seeds and enjoy.

Southwest Salad

What's inside:

Vinegar (1 Tbsp.)

Olive oil (2 tsp.)

Pepper

Salt

Cumin (.25 tsp.)

Chili powder (.5 tsp.)

Sweet kernel corn (1 c.)

Cubed avocado (1)

Cherry tomatoes (1 c.)

Chopped mixed greens (4 c.)

Sliced red bell pepper (1)

Diced purple onion (.5 c.)

Dry chickpeas (.5 c.)

Dry black beans (.5 c.)

How to make this:

1. You can go through and use your favorite method in order to get the chickpeas and black beans all ready to go.
2. When this is done, you can bring out a big bowl and add in all of the ingredients that we have above into it.
3. Toss the mix of spice and veggies together so they combine and mix well. store or serve chilled with a bit of vinegar and olive oil over it all.

Shaved Brussel Sprout Salad

What's inside

Dressing

Minced garlic (.5 Tbsp.)

Olive oil (2 Tbsp.)

Apple cider vinegar (2 Tbsp.)

Maple syrup (1 Tbsp.)

Brown mustard (1 Tbsp.)

For the Salad

Pepper

Salt

Dried cranberries (.5 c.)

Crushed walnuts (.5 c.)

Crushed almonds (.5 c.)

Sour apple (1)

Purple onion (1 c.)

Brussel sprouts (2 c.)

Dry chickpeas (.25 c.)

Red kidney beans, dry (.5 c.)

How to make this:

1. To start this recipe, start preparing the beans using one of your favorite methods.
2. When that is done, take out a bowl and combine together all of the ingredients that we are using for our dressing.
3. Add the dressing to the fridge and let it sit there for about an hour before you use it to serve.
4. When ready, you can take out a knife, mandolin, or grater and use it to thinly slice up your Brussel sprouts. You can repeat this same idea with the onion and the apple.
5. Now it is time to take out a big bowl and you can combine the nuts, cranberries, onions, apples, sprouts, beans, and chickpeas inside.
6. Sprinkle on some of the cold and prepared dressing to the salad and then serve with some pepper or salt to taste before enjoying.

***

Colorful Protein Power Salad

What's inside:

Pepper

Salt

Lemon juice (1 tsp.)

Olive oil (2 Tbsp.)

Shredded and chopped carrot (1 c.)

Chopped kale (4 c.)

Purple cabbage (3 c.)

Minced garlic (2 tsp.)

Chopped green onion (1)

Dry navy beans (2 c.)

Dry quinoa (.5 c.)

How to make this:

1. Take out the quinoa and then follow the directions on the box to figure out how to make it the right way. Then you are able to use your favorite methods in order to prepare the beans.
2. When ready, you can take out a frying pan and heat up about a tablespoon of olive oil.

3. When this is warm, you can add in the cabbage, garlic, and chopped green onion. Let this heat up for a few minutes.
4. Add in the rest of the oil with the salt and the kale and then lower the heat and cover this up until it is wilted.
5. After another five minutes of cooking this, you can take the pan off the stove and set it to the side.
6. Take out a big bowl here and then add in the rest of the ingredients with your prepared cabbage and kale mixture. Add in some more pepper and salt if you would like, mixing until it is all distributed in the right manner.
7. Serve this with some of the dressing on top of each serving and then enjoy right away.

***

Edamame and Ginger Citrus Salad

What's inside:

Dressing
Sesame oil (.5 Tbsp.)
Minced ginger (.5 tsp.)
Maple syrup (.5 Tbsp.)
Lime juice (1 tsp.)
Orange juice (.25 c.)

For the Salad

Sliced avocado (1)

Pepper

Salt

Chopped mint (2 tsp.)

Roasted sesame seeds (1 Tbsp.)

Shelled edamame (1 c.)

Chopped kale (4 c.)

Shredded carrots (2 c.)

Dry green lentils (.5 c.)

How to make this

1. Take out the lentils and then prepare them with the method that you like the most.
2. When that is done, you can bring out a bowl and combine the ginger, maple syrup, lime juices, and the orange juice. Mix up with a whisk while adding in your sesame oil slowly.
3. When that is done, take out another bowl and add in the mint, sesame seeds, edamame, kale, carrot, and the cooked lentils.
4. Add the dressing and then stir it all together as well as possible so that the ingredients can be coated in an even manner. Store or serve with some of the avocado and a bit more mint before serving.

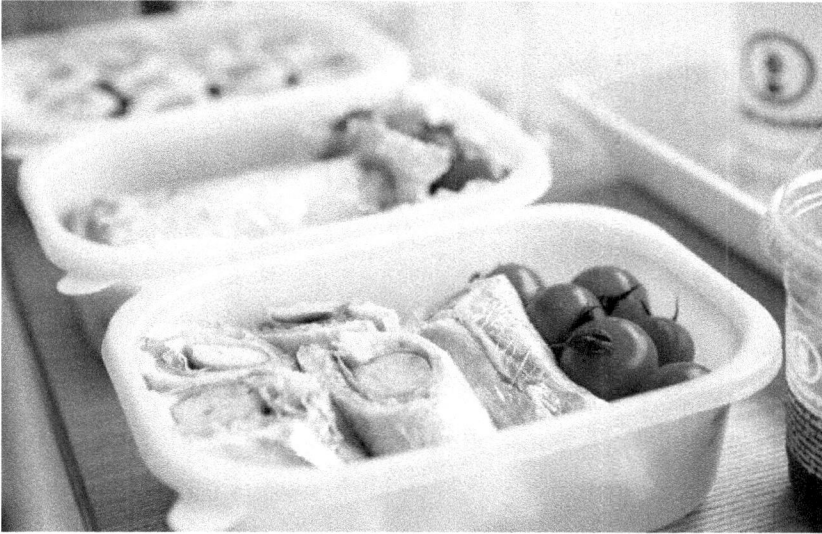

Vegan Mushroom Pho

What's inside

Pepper

Salt

Chopped cabbage (1 c.)

Chopped bok choy (1 c.)

Matchstick carrots (1 c.)

Raw bean sprouts (1 c.)

Rice noodles (2 c.)

Sesame oil (1 Tbsp.)

Hoisin sauce (2 Tbsp.)

Sliced mushrooms (3 c.)

Olive oil (1 Tbsp.)

Minced ginger (1 tsp.)

Sliced green onions (3)

Vegetable broth (6 c.)

Drained firm tofu (14 oz.)

How to make this:

1. Take the tofu out and cut into some cubes before setting to the side. Take out a pan and then heat up the vegetable broth along with the ginger and the green onions.
2. Boil this for a minute before reducing the heat to a low setting. Cover with the lid and then let it simmer for a bit.
3. After 20 minutes, take out another pan and heat up the oil. Add in the sliced mushrooms to the pan and cook until they become soft.
4. Then add in the sesame oil, hoisin sauce, and tofu. Heat up the sauce and let it get nice and thick. After 5 minutes, you can take this off the heat.
5. Use the instructions on the package of the noodles to prepare the rice noodles. Top these noodles with some of the tofu mushroom mixture and some broth and the bean sprouts.
6. Add in the carrots and then other ingredients as well if needed and then serve warm.

Ruby Red Burger

What's inside:

Buns (6)

Spinach, washed and dried (2 c.)

Pepper and salt

Onion powder (2 tsp.)

Chopped parsley (1 tsp.)

Balsamic vinegar (1 Tbsp.)

Garlic powder (2 Tbsp.)

Olive oil (2 Tbsp.)

Beets (2)

Dry quinoa (.5 c.)

Dry chickpeas (1 c.)

How to make this:

1. Start this recipe by heating up the oven to 400 degrees. Take the time to prepare the quinoa and the chickpeas according to the method that you prefer.
2. While those are getting prepared, you can peel and then dice up the beats and add them to a bowl along with the onion powder and the olive oil.

3. Spread out these beets in a baking pan and then add it to the oven. After 10 minutes, the beets should be done. You can then take them out of the oven to cool down.

4. When they are nice and cool, take the beets off the baking sheet and add them into the food processor along with the quinoa pepper garlic, parsley, salt vinegar, and chickpeas.

5. Pulse these ingredients for about half a minute to make them nice and crumble. Then you can use your hands to make six patties out of this mixture and add to a small pan.

6. Add these to the freezer for an hour until the patties are nice and firm. After that 60 minutes, take out a skillet and add in a bit of oil. Add the patties when it is warm.

7. These need to get browned on each side which can take about 4 minutes on both sides.

8. Serve these with a bit of spinach on the buns that you chose.

***

Mango and Tempeh Wraps

What's inside:

Salt (.25 tsp)

Lime juice (.25 tsp)

Garlic powder (1 Tbsp.)

Hoisin sauce (1 Tbsp.)

Sweet chili sauce (.25 c.)

Peeled and diced mangos (2)

Lettuce leaves (6)

Coconut oil (1 Tbsp.)

Tempeh (16 oz.)

How to make this:
1. Take out a big skillet and heat up some of the coconut oil on top. Cook the tempeh until it starts to crumble and is browned, making sure to stir it the whole time.
2. After about four minutes of cooking this, add in the salt, garlic, lime juice, and hoisin and heat it all the way through.
3. Slice up the mangoes into smaller cubes and then pour the sweet chili sauce into a bowl to mix with the cubes.
4. Scoop up your cooked tempeh and divide it up between the leaves of lettuce to use those as your wraps. Top with some of the mango chunks and then serve.

Creamy Squash Pizza

What's inside:

Sauce
Oregano (1 tsp.)

Paprika (1 tsp.)

Cumin (1 tsp.)

Red pepper flakes (1 tsp.)

Olive oil (1 Tbsp.)

Minced garlic (2 Tbsp.)

Cubed butternut squash (3 c.)

Crust
Onion powder (1 tsp.)

Italian seasoning (1 Tbsp.)

Minced garlic (2 Tbsp.)

Water (2 c.)

French green lentils (2 c.)

Toppings
Olive oil (1 Tbsp.)

Diced purple onion (1)

Diced head of broccoli (1)

Diced red bell pepper (1)

Diced green bell pepper (1)

How to make this:

1. Turn on the oven and give it some time to heat up to 350 degrees. While the oven is heating up, use your favorite method to heat up the French green lentils.
2. When you are ready, add all of the ingredients for the sauce into a food processor or blender and then blend on a low setting until all of this is mixed and the sauce starts to look creamy. Set this aside in a small bowl for now.
3. Clean out the food processor and then add in the ingredients that you are using for your crust. Pulse this at a high speed to make a batter that is like dough.
4. Heat up a deep-dish pan over your stove and grease it with just a bit of oil. Press this dough into the skillet to make it into a round pizza. When that is done, add to the oven to bake.
5. After a few minutes, about five you can put the crust onto a baking tray with some parchment paper and then top with the sauce and the rest of the toppings. Add to the oven to bake.
6. This needs to cook for around 15 minutes. When that time is up, take this out of the oven and slice up into four parts before serving.

***

Portobello Burgers

What's inside:

Salt

Chili powder (.5 tsp.)

Paprika (.5 tsp.)

Taco seasoning (1 Tbsp.)

Drained tofu (8 oz.)

Olive oil (1 Tbsp.)

Salsa (.25 c.)

Vegan buns (2)

Hummus (4 Tbsp.)

Red and green bell pepper, diced (.5 each)

Onion diced (.5)

Mushroom caps, portobello (4)

Spinach (3 c.)

How to make this:

1. Take the tofu and slice it up into four pieces. Then you can take out the skillet and warm up with some of the olive oil.
2. When this is warm, add in the mushrooms caps and then let them cook for four minutes before slipping them over. Sprinkle on the chili powder, taco seasoning, salt, and paprika.
3. Flip these again after another four minutes and then leave them to cook until they are about half their original size. When this is done, take them off the heat and set to the side.
4. Add your prepared slices of tofu and cook on both sides to make browned a bit and hen set to the side.
5. Now it is time to add both the peppers and the onion to the skillet. These need to cook for about 10 minutes so the vegetables can become brown.
6. When this happens, you can turn the heat down to a low setting and put the mushrooms back in to heat up.
7. While those are cooking, you can spread out the hummus on one side of your bun and then add the salsa to the other part. Top the hummus with a bit of the spinach.

8. Serve this with two of the tofu squares and two of the mushrooms, and as much of the vegetables as you would like and enjoy.

Sweet and Sour Tofu

What's inside

Drained tofu (14 oz)
Olive oil (2 Tbsp.)
Chopped red bell pepper (1)
Coconut sugar (1 Tbsp.)
Cornstarch (1 tsp.)
Minced garlic (.2 Tbsp>)
Diced white onion (1)
Minced ginger (.5-inch piece)
Cornstarch (1 tsp)
Soy sauce (2 Tbsp.)
Rice vinegar (2 Tbsp.)
Pineapple chunks (1 c.)
Tomato paste (1 Tbsp.)
Chopped green and red bell pepper (1 of each)

How to make this:

1. Take out a small bowl and then whisk together the sugar, cornstarch, vinegar, tomato paste and soy sauce.
2. Slice up the tofu into cubes and add into a bowl with the soy sauce mixture. Let this set to marinate the tofu for some time.
3. After the marinating is done, heat up a bit of the oil in a frying pan and when this is warm, add in the chunks of tofu and half of the marinade that is left into the pan. Let this cook.
4. After about 10 minutes, with lots of stirring in the process, you can take the tofu off the heat and let it set in a bowl.
5. Add the rest of the oil to the same pan and then put the garlic and ginger inside. Heat this up for a minute before adding in the peppers and onion. Cook these to help the vegetables get nice and soft.
6. After another 5 minutes, you can pour the rest of the marinade into the pan with the vegetables and let these heat up until the sauce can get thick.
7. Add in the tofu cubes and the pineapple chunks and cook to heat up before serving.

***

BBQ Sliders

What's inside:

Tomatoes, pickles, onions for topping
Asian style slaw for topping
Slider buns (6)
Onion powder (1 tsp.)
Garlic powder (1 tsp.)
BBQ sauce (.5 c.)
Green jackfruit (2 cans)

How to make:

1. Bring out a big bowl and use a fork or your own potato masher to help get the jackfruit mashed to a shredded type of consistency.
2. Heat up a stockpot and add in the onion powder, garlic powder, BBQ sauce, and shredded jackfruit.
3. Stir this around and cover the pot. After 10 minutes, then you can take the lid off.
4. If you notice that the jackfruit is starting to stick then you can add in a bit of water or vegetable broth to help with this.
5. When the lid is off, you can cook for a few more minutes to heat all the way up.

6. Serve this on some of the slider buns and add on your favorite toppings before serving.

Hawaiian Burgers

What's inside:

Toppings of your choice
Buns (8)
Pineapple sliced into rings (1)
Onion powder (1 tsp.)
Garlic powder (1 tsp.)
Pineapple juice (.25 c.)
BBQ sauce (.25 c.)
Oats that are quick cooking (1 .c)
Cooked brown rice (2 c.)
Cooked black beans (3 c.)

How to make:

1. Turn on the grill at the beginning of this and get it up to medium-high heat.
2. In the meantime, take out a bowl and use a fork to help mash the black beans in. then add in the onion powder, garlic powder, pineapple juice, BBQ sauce, oats, and rice into it.

3. Combine this mixture until it is able to hold its own shape and can be formed into patties.

4. Scoop out about half a cup of this and form into a patty. Repeat to use up the whole mixture and then add these onto the grill.

5. Cook for about 5 minutes on the one side and then flip them over to cook on that side.

6. Add the pineapple rings on the grill at this time and only cook for a few minutes on each side.

7. When this is done, take the pineapple rings and burgers off the grill. Add one pineapple ring and one patty onto each bun.

8. Top with some of the BBQ sauce and some of the favorite toppings you chose before serving.

***

Falafel Burgers

What's inside:

Favorite toppings
Whole-wheat buns or pita pockets
Ground pepper (.25 tsp.)
Ground coriander (1 tsp.)
Ground cumin (1.5 tsp.)
Onion powder (2 tsp.)
Garlic powder (2 tsp.)
Lemon juice (1 Tbsp.)
Chopped parsley that is fresh (.25 c.)
Vegetable broth (.25 c.)
Brown rice that is cooked (2 c.)
Cooked chickpeas (3 c.)

How to make:

1. Turn on the oven and let it heat up to 425 degrees. While the oven is heating up you can take out a baking sheet and line with some parchment paper.
2. Now bring out your food processor and combine the pepper, coriander, onion powder, cumin, garlic powder, lemon juice, parsley, broth, rice, and chickpeas.

3. Process these ingredients together for about half a minute. You don't want it to turn into hummus but have it enough so that it forms into patties.
4. When this is done take about half a cup of the mixture and form it into patties. Add onto your prepared baking sheet and then repeat that with the rest of the mixture.
5. Add this to the oven and let it bake. After 15 minutes, take these out of the oven and then flip them around before cooking for another 15 minutes.
6. When this is done, take the patties out of the oven to cool down. Fill up the buns or the pitas with some of your favorite toppings and then add in the burgers to serve.

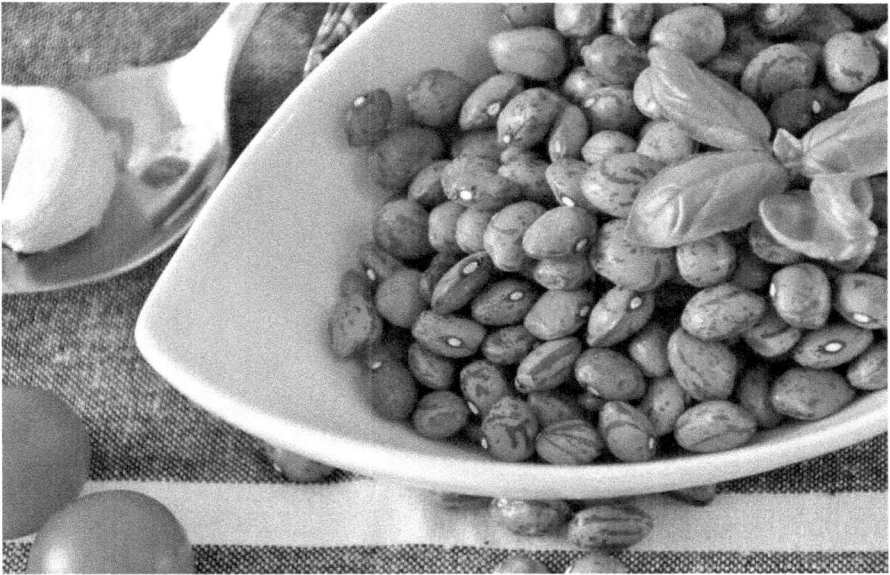

Black Bean and Quinoa Burgers

What's inside:

Roasted sesame seeds

Lettuce leaves (4)

Pepper (1 tsp.)

Salt (1 tsp.)

Dry black beans (1 .c)

Dry quinoa (.5 c.)

Chopped purple onion (.5)

Paprika (.5 tsp.)

Olive oil (2 Tbsp.)

Red pepper flakes (.5 tsp.)

Minced garlic (2 Tbsp.)

Whole wheat flour (.5 c.)

Chopped bell pepper (.25 c.)

How to make this:

1. Start out this recipe by preparing the beans using your favorite method. You can also take this time to prepare the quinoa-based on the instructions on the back of the box.
2. When you are ready, heat up a bit of olive oil in a frying pan and when it is nice and hot, add in the onions, bell peppers, and garlic and then season with some pepper and salt.
3. Cook these until you are able to get the vegetables to soften, which can take around five minutes. When that time is done, take the pan from the heat and let them cool down.
4. When these are all cooled down, which can take around 10 minutes, you can add the vegetables to the food processor along with the rest of the spices, the quinoa, flour, and cooked beans Pulse to make this into a chunky mixture.

5. Take out a pan and cover it with some parchment paper. Form this mixture into four patties and then add to the freezer for the next five minutes to help them stick together better.

6. When that time is up, add the rest of the oil to a frying pan and heat it up. When the pan is warm, add the patties inside.

7. Cook these until all of the sides are browned, which will take about 3 minutes on aside. Serve these with a burger bun or lettuce leaf and some of your favorite toppings.

***

Stuffed Peppers

What's inside:

Pepper

Salt

Dry black beans (1 c.)

Dry chickpeas (.5 c.)

Kale (.5 c)

Parsley (1 Tbs.)

Water (2 Tbsp.)

Olive oil (2 Tbsp.)

Bell peppers, any color (3)

Dry quinoa (.5 co

Sweet onion, chopped (1)

Garlic, minced (2 Tbsp.)

How to make this:

1. Start out by preparing the beans by following your favorite method. You can also go through and prepare the quinoa using the directions that are on the package.
2. In the meantime, you can heat up the oven and let it get to 400 degrees. While that is heating up, you can slice up the bell peppers and get rid of the stem and the seeds.
3. Add these to the baking sheet, making sure to have the skin down, and add on a bit of the oil to them. Add to the oven
4. After about 10 minutes, the skin on the peppers should be softening and it is time to take them out and let them cool down.
5. While your peppers are in the oven add some oil to a pan and heat it up. Add in the onion and let it cook for a few minutes before stirring in the water, parsley, kale, garlic, and basil.
6. Cook all of these together for a few more minutes before adding in the prepared chickpeas, quinoa, and black beans, warming them all the way through.
7. Spoon this mixture into the cooked pepper halves and then put all of this back into the oven to heat up.
8. After another 10 minutes, you can take the bell peppers out of the oven and let them cool down before serving.

Sweet Potato Sushi

What's inside:

Tamari (1 Tbsp)
Silken tofu (14 oz.)
Nori sheets (4)
Agave nectar (1 Tbsp.)
Rice vinegar (1 Tbsp.)
Dry sushi rice (.75 c)
Peeled sweet potato (1)
Sliced avocado (1)
Water (1 c)

How to make this:

1. Turn on the oven and give it time to heat up to 400 degrees. While that is warming up, take the tamari and mix it together with the agave nectar until they are combined together well and then set to the side.
2. Next, we need to slice up the sweet potato into sticks and place them onto a prepared baking sheet. Coat them with some of the agave and tamari mixtures. Add to the oven.

3. Bake these in the oven until they get nice and soft, making sure to flip them around during the cooking process as well.

4. After 25 minutes, these will be done. In the meantime, bring out a pot and add the vinegar, water, and the sushi rice inside. Bring this to a boil and let it cook until most of the liquid is gone, which will take around ten minutes.

5. While we are cooking the rice, we can cut up the tofu into long sticks and set aside. Take the pot off the heat when they are done and let the rice sit for about 10 minutes.

6. Cover up the work surface that you are using with some parchment paper and wet your fingers. Layout the nori sheet on here and add a thin layer of the rice. Leave some room to roll up the sheet.

7. Add the strips of roasted sweet potato on here in a straight line and then lay the avocado and tofu slices right beside them as well.

8. When this is done, you can roll up the nori sheet into a tight cylinder. Slice this into 8 pieces and then put it in the fridge. Repeat with the rest of the nori sheets and fillings.

9. Serve this chilled and enjoy.

***

Sweet Potato Chili

What's inside:

Chopped parsley
Pepper
Salt
Olive oil (1 Tbsp.)
Water (.5 c)
Cayenne (.5 tsp.)
Paprika (.5 tsp.)
Chili powder (1 Tbsp.)
Red bell pepper (.5)
Cumin (1 tsp.)
Green bell pepper (.5)
Tofu, (14 oz.)
Diced tomatoes with green chilies (1 can)
Sweet potatoes, cubed (2)
Diced onion, sweet (1)

How to make this:

1. To start this recipe, take out a pot and heat up some of the olive oil inside. When that is warm, add in the garlic and onions and let them cook until they are nice and soft.
2. When this is done, add in the bell peppers and stir to make it all nice and tender, which can take another five minutes.
3. When five minutes is up, you can reduce the heat to low and then add in all of your remaining ingredients. Stir this around to combine well and let it cook.
4. After another 20 minutes, the sweet potatoes should be soft and the liquid should be nice and thick.
5. Serve this in a warm bowl and enjoy!

***

Coconut Tofu Curry

What's inside:

Pepper

Salt

Firm tofu (14 oz.)

Agave nectar (1 tsp.)

Coconut oil (2 tsp.)

Red pepper flakes (.5 tsp.)

Can of coconut milk (13 oz.)

Cumin (1 tsp.)

Diced tomatoes (1)

Curry powder (1 tsp.)

Turmeric (1 tsp.)

Snap peas (1 c.)

Ginger, minced

How to make this:

1. To start this recipe, slice the tofu into smaller cubes. Then take out a skillet and heat up the coconut oil inside to make it hot.

2. When the oil is nice and warm, add in the tofu and let it cook for a bit. After 5 minutes, add in the onion and garlic and cook for another five minutes before adding in the ginger as well.

3. When that is nice and warmed up, it is time to add in the rest of the spices along with the snap peas, tomatoes, coconut milk, and agave nectar.

4. Combine well and then cover up the pot cooking this on low heat. After another 10 minutes, you can take the whole pot off the heat.

5. When you are ready to serve, scoop this prepared curry onto some rice or into a bowl and enjoy it.

***

Tahini Falafels

What's inside:

Tahini (2 Tbsp.)

Salt

Turmeric (.25 tsp.)

Paprika (.5 tsp.)

Lemon juice (.5 tsp.)

Olive oil (1 tsp.)

Cumin (2 tsp.)

Minced garlic clove (1)

Broccoli florets (2 c.)

Black beans dry (.5 c.)

Dry chickpeas (2 c.)

How to make this:

1. You can go through and cook up the black beans and the chickpeas by following the method that you want to use.
2. While those are cooking, you can turn on the oven to 400 degrees and let it get warm.
3. Take out a skillet and drizzle some broccoli florets with the oil and salt. Add the broccoli to the warm skillet and let them cook to become brown and tender. This should be done after ten minutes.
4. When that is done, move the broccoli off the heat and let it cool down. Add this prepared broccoli into the food processor with all of your ingredients besides the tahini and blend until it is smooth and most of the lumps are gone.
5. Take out a baking pan and add some parchment paper to it. Press the dough that you just made into 8 patties that are equal and then place them on the parchment paper. Add to the oven.
6. Bake these until they are crisp and brown on the outside, which can take around 15 minutes. Make sure that you flip these around about halfway through so that the cooking is even as possible.
7. Serve with the tahini as a topping and enjoy.

***

Baked Enchilada

What's inside:

Vegan cheese (.5 c.)

Salt (1 tsp.)

Garlic powder (1 tsp)

Paprika (1 tsp.)

Chopped cashews (.5 c.)

Cumin (1 tsp.)

Firm tofu (14 oz.)

Diced purple onion (.5)

Green pepper (1)

Enchilada sauce (2 c.)

Olive oil (4 Tbsp.)

Sweet potato (1)

Black beans (1 c.)

Chopped jalapenos (1 Tbsp.)

How to make this

1. Turn on the oven and let it heat up to 400 degrees. While that is warming up, take the sweet potatoes and slice them into cubes before adding to a big bowl.

2. Top with a bit of the olive oil, the salt, and the garlic powder. Toss these around so that the sweet potatoes will be coated as evenly as possible.

3. When this is done, add to the prepared baking pan and then put them in the oven to cook until they are soft. This will take around 20 minutes.

4. While those are baking, dice up the tofu onion and bell pepper into small cubes and then place into the bowl with the salt, cashews, and olive oil. Stir these well to make sure it is all coated evenly.

5. When the potatoes are done, add the onion, peppers, and tofu to the baking pan and then stir to combine. Add all of these back into the oven to bake for a bit.

6. After ten minutes the peppers should be soft and the onions brown. Take these out of the oven and then place it into a casserole dish.

7. Add the black beans, spices, and the enchilada sauce to the dish and mix to make sure it is all combined. Top with your vegan cheese before adding back into the oven to bake.

8. After another 15 minutes, this should be done. Take out of the oven and give it some time to cool down. Top with the jalapenos and then serve.

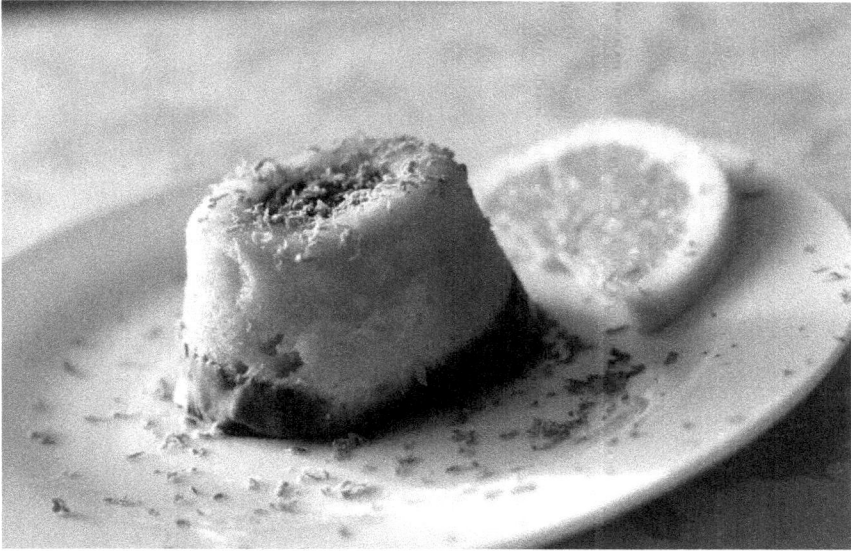

Energy Crackers

What's inside:

Pepper

Salt

Flax seeds (.25 c.)

Chia seeds (.25 c.)

Paprika powder (.25 tsp.)

Sesame seeds (.25 c)

Water (.75 c.)

Minced garlic (1 Tbsp.)

Cashews crushed (.25 c.)

Crushed peanuts (.25 c.)

Dried onion flakes (.5 Tbsp.)

Pumpkin seeds (.5 c)

How to make this

1. To start this recipe, turn on the oven and let it heat up to 350 degrees. While the oven is heating up, take out a big bowl and combine the onion flakes, water, garlic, and paprika. Mix together well.

2. To that same bowl, you will want to add the chia seeds, sesame seeds, pumpkin seeds, cashews, peanuts, and flax seeds.

3. Stir all of this together well but add in some pepper and salt to your own preferences here.

4. When that is done, take out a baking sheet and line with some parchment paper. Spread out this mixture and then add it to the heated oven.

5. After 25 minutes, these should be done. Take them out of the oven and then flip it over so that it is easier to cut.

6. Slice into as many squares as you would like and then put it back into the oven to finish baking.

7. After another half an hour, these crackers are done. Allow them to have some time cooling down before serving.

***

Chocolate and Zucchini Muffins

What's inside:

Water (.5 c.)

Salt

Nutmeg (.5 tsp.)

Vanilla (.5 tsp.)

Cinnamon (.5 tsp.)

Baking powder (2 tsp.)

Almond milk 5 Tbsp.)

Dark chocolate chips (.5 c.)

Chocolate protein powder (1 c.)

Shredded zucchini (.5 c.)

Maple syrup (.25 c.)

Applesauce (.5 c.)

Banana (2)

Chopped walnuts (.5 c.)

Almond flour (1.5 c.)

Coconut oil (2 Tbsp.)

Dry quinoa (.5 c.)

How to make this:

1. Take the time to follow the directions on the back of the box to cook up and prepare the quinoa that we are using.
2. Turn on the oven and give it time to heat up to 400 degrees. While that is getting nice and warm, prepare a muffin pan with some coconut oil and set to the side.
3. Now we need to take out a big bowl and mix together the baking powder, cinnamon, walnuts, salt, nutmeg, flour, and prepared quinoa.
4. Then bring out a second bowl and mash together the bananas with a fork. Combine these with the applesauce.
5. Stir in the almond milk, protein powder, maple syrup, and vanilla until they are distributed well, adding in some more water if it is needed.
6. Combine these two separate mixtures into one bowl and then stir to make sure the batter is all smooth. Then finally fold in the chocolate chips and the shredded zucchini.
7. Take the batter and fill up the muffin cups to the halfway point. Then add these to the oven to bake.
8. After 20 minutes, you can take these out of the oven and let them cool down a bit before serving or storing.

***

Lemon Pie Bars

What's inside:

Salt (.25 tsp.)
Lemon juice (2 Tbsp.)
Protein powder, vanilla (.5 c.)
Pitted dates (2 c.)
Sunflower seeds (.33 c.)
Raw cashews (.33 c.)
Pecan pieces (.25 c.)
Chia seeds (.25 c.)

How to make this:

1. Take some time before we start to soak our chia seeds in some water. Drain out the water that is left when you are done.
2. Take out the food processor next and then place the sunflower seeds, chia seeds, pecans, and cashews inside. Let these pulse on a low setting until you get a crumbly mixture out of it.
3. Now it is time to add the dates, lemon juice, and salt and then continue to pulse while you add in some of the protein powder so you get a chunky kind of dough.

4. Add this o a baking sheet that has some parchment paper on it. Press this out using a rolling pin to get a nice thick square.
5. Add this to the freezer to get it to set, for about 60 minutes. When the chunk is solid you can slice into 8 pieces and enjoy.

***

Spicy Chickpea Poppers

What's inside:

Cayenne pepper (.25 tsp.)
Paprika (.25 tsp.)
Cumin (.25 tsp.)
Onion powder (.25 tsp.)
Garlic powder (.5 tsp.)
Chili powder (.5 tsp.)
Salt (.5 tsp.)
Coconut oil (1 Tbsp.)
Chickpeas (2 c.)

How to make this:

1. Take some time to cook the chickpeas according to the method that you like the most.
2. When those are done, you can turn on the oven and let it heat up to 400 degrees. While the oven is getting warm, use some parchment paper to line the baking sheet.
3. Add the chickpeas when they are done to a big plate and then pat them dry. Add to the baking sheet before coating with the garlic powder, onion powder, salt, and coconut oil.
4. Add these to the oven so the chickpeas can bake. When they are fragrant and brown, which will take around half an hour, then you can take them out of the oven.
5. Allow the chickpeas some time to cool down and then add them to a bowl. Mix with the rest of the spices that we have not used yet until coated well and then serve warm.

***

Almond Protein Bars

What's inside:

Coconut oil (1 tsp.)

Applesauce (2 Tbsp.)

Flax seeds (.25 c.)

Chopped almonds (.25 c)

Dried cranberries (.25 c.)

Pitted dates (.5 c.)

Chocolate protein powder (.5 c.)

Almond butter (1 c)

How to make this

1. Take out a baking dish and line it with some parchment paper before setting it to the side.
2. Add all of your ingredients into the setup the food processor and then blend them together to make a thick dough.
3. Press this prepared dough into your baking dish, making sure here to properly press it into each corner. You can use your hands to make sure this is pressed down as well as possible throughout the whole pan.

4. Add this to the fridge to set for about two hours. If you need it done a bit faster, add to the freezer and chill for an hour.

5. Slice into 8 bars and then enjoy or serve right away.

***

Matcha Energy Balls

What's inside:

Maple syrup (1 Tbsp.)

Matcha powder (1 Tbsp.)

Raw cashews (1 c.)

Pistachios (.5 c.)

Crushed hazelnuts (.25 c.)

Coconut, shredded (.25 c.)

Vanilla protein powder (.5 c.)

Packed and pitted dates (.5 c.)

How to make this:

1. Bring out a food processor and get it all set up nicely. Add in all of the ingredients outside of the hazelnuts to the food processor and then blend on low to make it all combined and crushed well.

2. When this is done, bring out a spoon and scoop out heaps of this mixture. Use your own hands along the way in order to roll into balls.

3. Pour the hazelnuts, after they are crushed, into a bowl and then roll the matcha balls into the hazelnuts until they are coated all around.

4. Add these, when they are all coated, into the fridge and let them sit there until they are solid. This will take about half an hour to finish and then serve!

***

Black Bean Dip

What's inside:

Salt (.25 tsp.)
Lemon juice (1 Tbsp.)
Olive oil (1 Tbsp.)
Onion powder (2 Tbsp.)
Italian seasoning (2 Tbsp.)
Minced garlic (2 Tbsp.)
Cooked black beans (4 c.)

How to make this:

1. Take all of the black beans and add them into a bowl. Mash these up with a fork until you get them to be pretty smooth.
2. When this is done, you can stir in the rest of the ingredients and incorporate them well. you want to make sure this mixture is as creamy and smooth as possible.
3. Add in some more lemon juice and salt to taste if you would like and then serve at room temperature.

Sunflower Protein Bars

What's inside:

Salt (.25 tsp.)

Nutmeg (.25 tsp.)

Cinnamon (1 tsp.)

Vanilla (2 tsp.)

Sunflower butter (.5 c.)

Maple syrup (.5 c)

Chocolate protein powder (1 c.)

Rice cereal puffy (1 c.)

Old fashioned oats (1 c.)

How to make this:

1. Take out a big bowl and mix together the salt, nutmeg, cinnamon, protein powder, rice cereal, and oats. Set this to the side.

2. In a second bowl, you are able to add in the maple syrup and the sunflower butter and heat it up in the microwave for about half a minute.

3. When this is done, take it out of the microwave and then add it to the bowl with the dry ingredients. Stir these together well until you have a mixture that is smooth and no lumps are present.

4. Spread this mixture out into a shallow dish that has some parchment paper and then pack it down inside firmly. Use a spoon if needed to help get rid of the air bubbles.
5. Move this dish to the freezer and then let it set in there for about 20 minutes. When this is done, take the dish back out and slice into 6 parts before enjoying it.

***

Cake Batter Smoothie

What's inside:

Nutmeg (.25 tsp.)
Vanilla (1 tsp.)
Cinnamon (1 tsp.)
Cashew butter (1 Tbsp.)
Chocolate protein powder (4 Tbsp.)
Quick oats (.25 c.)
Almond milk (1 c.)
Banana (1)

How to make this:

1. Bring out a small jar or bowl and mix together the almond milk and your oats.
2. Add this into the fridge to give the oats some time to soften. Usually, this will need around an hour to complete.
3. After this time, add the milk and oats mixture into the blender with the rest of the ingredients.
4. Blend this on high speed until you have it all smooth and the lumps are all gone. Serve in some tall glasses with a bit of cinnamon on top and enjoy.

***

Protein Trail Mix Bars

What's inside:

Salt (.25 tsp.)

Cinnamon (.25 tsp.)

Chocolate protein powder (.5 c.)

Maple syrup (.25 c.)

Raw walnuts (1 c.)

Pecan halves (2 c.)

Raw almonds (2 c.)

How to make this:

1. Heat up a frying pan and when it is nice and warm, add in the protein powder, maple syrup, and nuts.
2. Stir this constantly so that the ingredients are going to turn into a thick and tacky kind of mixture. This can take up to ten minutes.
3. When that time is done, it is time to sprinkle on the cinnamon and salt over this and then cook for another few minutes.
4. When this is done, line a shallow pan with some parchment paper and then spread out the nut mixture onto it. Spread this out well and then give it some time to cool down all of the ways.
5. When you are ready to serve, you can go through and slice into 8 pieces before serving.

Mocha Chocolate Brownie Bars

What's inside:

Cold-brewed coffee (1 c)

Agave nectar (2 Tbsp.)

Nutmeg (.25 tsp.)

Vanilla (1 tsp.)

Quick oats (.5 c.)

Cocoa powder (.5 c)

Chocolate protein powder (2.5 c)

How to make this:

1. Take out a baking dish and line it with a bit of parchment paper. Set it to the side.
2. When that is done, take out a bowl and mix together the dry ingredients. Slowly add in the cold coffee, vanilla, and agave nectar, making sure to stir the whole time so that the lumps in the mixture are going to disappear.
3. When you have gotten rid of all the lumps, pour this batter into your prepared dish, making sure to press it down in all of the corners.
4. Now it is time to add the dish to the fridge to set until firm. This can take about four hours, or move it to the freezer and let it sit for about an hour.
5. Slice this into 6 even squares and then serve.

Cherry Vanilla Protein Bars

What's inside:

Vanilla (1 Tbsp.)
Almond milk (1 Tbsp.)
Chia seeds (.25 c.)
Maple syrup (.25 c)
Dried cranberries (.5 c.)
Cashew butter (.4 c)
Shredded coconut (.33 c.)
Vanilla protein powder (2 c.)
Oats (1 c.)

How to make this:

1. To start this recipe, take out a baking dish and line it with some parchment paper before setting it to the side.
2. When that is done, take out a blender and add in the coconut, protein powder, and oats inside. You will want to blend this until they are in a nice fine powder.
3. When this one is done, move it to a big bowl and then add in the rest of the ingredients that you are using. Mix well with a spoon until it is thoroughly combined.

4. Move this dough into a baking dish and then press down with your hands until you are able to get it to be as even as possible.
5. Place this into the freezer so that it has time to get firm. This will take around an hour and a half.
6. When that time is done, take it out of the freezer and slice into 8 bars before serving.

***

Banana and Peanut Butter Cookies

What's inside:

Salt (1 pinch)

Cocoa nibs (1 Tbsp.)

Nutmeg (.25 tsp.)

Cinnamon (.5 tsp.)

Vanilla (1 Tbsp.)

Ground flaxseed (1 Tbsp.)

Baking powder (1 Tbsp.)

Chocolate protein powder (.5 c.)

Maple syrup (.25 c.)

Chopped peanuts (.25 c)

Chunky peanut butter (.5 c.)

Banana (1)

Dry chickpeas (1 c.)

How to make this:

1. You can go through and prepare the chickpeas using the method you like the best.
2. When those are done, turn on the oven and let it heat up to 375 degrees. Then take out a baking pan and line it with a bit of parchment paper before setting it to the side.
3. Continue to add the cooked chickpeas and the other ingredients besides the cocoa nibs, to your food processor. Pulse these on a low setting until you see the mixture is getting nice and smooth.
4. When that is done, move it to a big bowl and then nicely stir in the cocoa nibs that you are using.
5. Now it is time to take a spoon and spoon the batter you made onto the baking pan. Press down on the batter a bit to get even baking. Add the pan to the oven to bake.
6. After about 8 to 10 minutes, the cookies should be done. Take them out of the oven to cool down before serving warm.

CONCLUSION

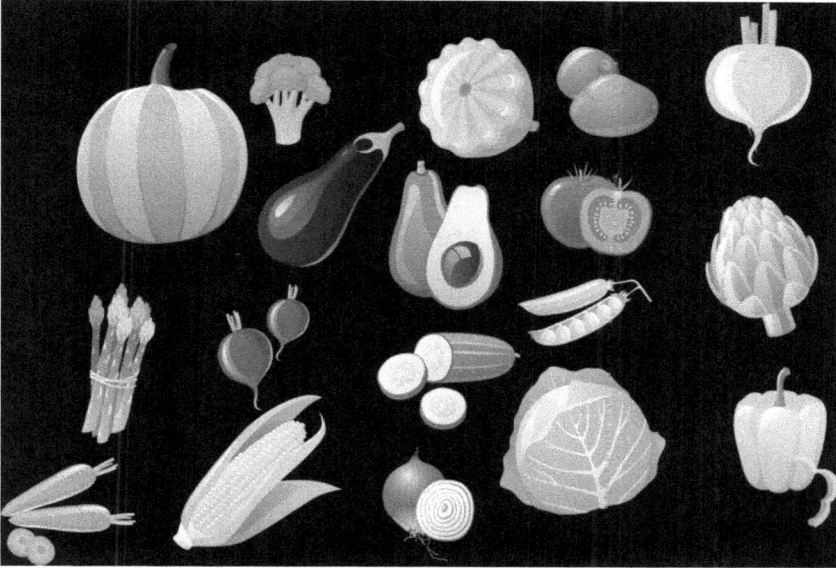

Thank you for making it through to the end of *Vegan Meal Prep for Beginners*, let's hope it was informative and able to provide you with all of the tools you need to achieve your goals whatever they may be.

The next step is to get started using the vegan diet plan. This is one of the best options that you are able to work with, and there are so many health benefits that you can get when you follow this diet, much more than you will find with any other diet plan out there. And when we are able to combine it together with some of the great tips and suggestions that come with meal prepping, you will find that it is easier than ever to get all of the nutrients and health that you are looking for along the way.

This guidebook took the time to look more into how we can work with meal planning to make the vegan diet to make things a whole lot easier in the process. When we are able to make the meal plan easier so that we are able to go on the vegan diet without a lot of problems at all. That is what this guidebook is going to take a look at and this can help you to lose a lot of weight and so much more.

There are a lot of benefits to following the vegan diet, and working with some meal planning along with it can make life so much easier overall. When you are ready to work with the vegan diet and meal planning together to make life easier, make sure to check out this guidebook to get started.

Finally, if you found this book useful in any way, a review on Amazon is always appreciated!